Leave Depression Behind

Let God Heal Your Heart While You Heal Your Habits

What Readers are Saying about *Leave Depression Behind*

"As one addicted to pleasing people, I found the raw honesty of this book refreshing. Vicki Huffman gives us permission to reject the judgment of others while choosing a victory much bigger than our circumstances."

– Bill Stanley, Nomad Pastor

"Any type of depression is tough. It can bring you to a snapping point. Use the tools in this book, because Vicki Huffman gives the best advice I've heard. Trust in our God. Speak to him daily. Great read!"

– Kelly LeStarge, Sadness to Joy Member

"Huffman shares her 40-year journey from depression to clarity. After pulling herself out of the muck and mire, she has a heart to help others escape, too. Easy read with great exercises to start documenting your own journey to wellness and joy. This book will be a lighthouse to many who have suffered far too long."

– Rhonda Bolling, Children's Book Author
www.rhondabolling.com

"Tired of carrying the unbearable weight of grief, trauma, failure, and approval-seeking? In *Leave Depression Behind*, Huffman shares from her own life experience how to change our thinking and habits and let God guide us through each day and each challenge. It's time to say, 'No more' and leave depression behind."

– Daniel Walker – pastor, activist, and
founder of Camino Road

Leave Depression Behind

Let God Heal Your Heart While You Heal Your Habits

Vicki Huffman

Sadness to Joy Publications
a division of Sadness to Joy Ministries

SADNESS TO JOY
MINISTRIES

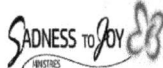

Leave Depression Behind
Copyright © 2019 by Vicki Huffman

Book Design by Vicki Huffman

Printed in the United States of America
First printing November, 2019

ISBN-13: 978-0-9988954-1-3

Dedication

I dedicate this book to all those who have missed even a single day of a joy-filled life because they were suffering from depression. I can't tell my story without telling of the saving grace of Jesus Christ, the countless hours of help I received from Dr. Astrid Sande and Kelly Jo Kaye, LMHC, and the unconditional love and support I received from my husband and family. I could not have persevered through this difficult journey without each of you.

May God Bless Your Journey to Joy.

Contents

Introduction   11

PART I How Did I Get Here?

1   I (Don't) Need to Stay Where It's Safe   17
2   I (Don't) Need Everyone to Like Me   31
3   I (Don't) Need to Do Everything Right   41
4   I (Don't) Need to Be in Control   51

PART II How Do I Get Help?

5   I Need to Admit I Need Help   65
6   I Need to Understand I'm Never Alone   75
7   I Need to Ask Those Who Know   95
8   I Need to Accept Help   107

PART III How Do I Get Better?

9   I Need to See Things Differently   119
10   I Need to Learn How to Breathe   131
11   I Need to Live in the Moment   147
12   I Need a New Direction   159
13   I Need to Count My Blessings   175

PART IV How Do I Help Others?

14   I Need to Help Others   189
15   I Need to Change My Focus   197
Notes   209
Who Am I   211
About the Author   215
Also by Vicki Huffman   217

Introduction

I Have Depression – Now What?

You may have picked up this book because you feel like you have depression. You may have even been diagnosed with depression. Or you may have a loved one who suffers from depression. Whatever brought you here, let me assure you, I understand. I've been there.

Because I've been there, I have an idea what you may be feeling. I certainly can't understand it completely. No one can. However, only someone who's been there before can begin to try.

I want to try.

I want to understand.

And I want to help.

This book was written out of my pain. The pain I experienced through forty years of depression. The pain I no longer experience. I've been able to leave my depression behind, and you can do the same. However, it won't be easy.

It's a task that will require:

- An all-in commitment

- Continuous self-examination

- Daily action focused on changing habits

- Endless reflection

This is a personal journey. No two people who take it will be the same.

We all start from different places. What worked for me may not work for you; but it's a good place to start.

Once you've started on the road to recovery, you'll discover what works best for you. You can then tweak your plan to provide the best chance of success. While having a plan is great, it's the amount of effort you put in that will determine your success on this journey and whether you reach the finish line. I have faith in you. I know you can do it.

How Can This Book Help Me?

This book is divided into four parts. It takes you on a journey through the four stages of recovery I personally went through. It is meant to accomplish two things: to help you understand you're not alone and to provide inspiration and hope that you, too, can leave depression behind.

As we walk through the journey I took, we'll explore four questions:

- How did I get here?

- How do I get help?

- How do I get better?

- How do I help others?

Each chapter will explore a portion of my journey combined with truth from God's Word. The truth about what I needed and what I didn't need to move forward. The truth that set me free from depression.

Inspirational Suggestions

In each chapter, I've included a few scriptures, quotes, and/or songs that helped me. They are meant to encourage and inspire you to make the positive changes needed to overcome your depression. Take time to memorize them and/or use them as positive affirmations. (*Links have been shortened using bitly.com*)

Reflection

At the end of each chapter, I've included some questions for personal reflection. Yes, this book is about my journey. However, that's not all. It's meant to inspire you to take your own journey. It's also meant to help you document your journey as you leave depression behind.

Forcing yourself to answer the reflection questions will ensure you've not just read the chapter, but you've processed the truth of it and how it can apply to your life.

Ready to Get Started?

Only you can decide if it's time to leave your depression behind. If you aren't sure you're strong enough to do the hard work needed, that's okay. As I said, this book is meant to inspire and encourage you to take that journey. When you're ready, when you've decided you don't want to live like you have been anymore, you'll find the strength to do what it takes. In the meantime, take comfort as you discover you aren't alone. There is hope.

PART I

How Did I Get Here?

1

I (Don't) Need to Stay Where It's Safe

An Honest Look at What Safety Costs

How far can you stretch a rubber band? That depends on the rubber band. You must consider its overall strength and the resistance it is built to withstand. Rubber bands can be designed to hold your braces in place or your hair in a ponytail. Others are strong enough to hold a stack of folders stuffed full of papers. Each can withstand a different amount of stretching before it will break. This is called tensile strength—the largest amount of force that can be applied to an object being stretched or pulled before it breaks.[1]

Our emotions have a tensile strength as well. Have your emotions ever been overwhelmed, raw, and stretched to the limit? Then, with no warning—SNAP! The symbolic rubber band that held your emotions together suddenly broke, creating chaos out of order and hurting anyone in its path.

Throughout my life, I lived under the misguided belief I could stretch the limit of my emotions without consequences. I'd stretch myself right up to the breaking point and then ease the tension just enough to breathe. Then I'd stretch right back up to that limit again. My life was a seemingly endless emotional-tensile-strength challenge.

Until that day!

On October 29, 2014, I snapped. In the same way a rubber band explodes into pieces when, without warning, it reaches that invisible breaking point, my life was shattered. The contents of my neat and orderly life, which had previously been held together ever so fragilely, lay shattered before me.

With nothing left of what I knew as normal, I was forced to start over, to take an honest look at my personal circumstances, my thoughts, and my beliefs. It was time to conduct an authentic investigation into why I'd made the choices I had throughout my life, which had gotten me to this point. I needed to answer the question, *How in the world did I get here?*

An Honest Look at My Circumstances

We've all had different experiences in life that have led us to where we are today: looking at how to survive depression. I know what you're going through because I've already been there. Fortunately, I've come out on the other side strong enough to know I don't want anyone else to go through what I did. Experience truly is the best teacher.[2]

So, how did I get here? For me, it was post-traumatic stress disorder (PTSD). Interestingly enough, it wasn't actually the traumatic event that caused my depression. It was forty years of acting like it hadn't happened. It was forty years of failing to ask for help. That's right, I simply failed to ask for help.

I knew I needed help, and I know people would have gladly helped me if I'd only asked. Sadly, I was just too ashamed to admit it. I was too ashamed to ask. Why was admitting I needed help so hard?

It was hard because of my strict upbringing. I grew up in the church. We were there several times a week. I knew all the Bible stories and the words to a ton of hymns (all five verses). I was baptized at the age of thirteen, as was the custom in our church. I knew Jesus loved me and had died for my sins. I also knew what it meant to follow Jesus.

Yet all that head knowledge didn't mean I really knew Jesus in my heart and soul. What it meant was every Sunday morning I put on my best clothing and was on my best behavior.

With that strong faith background, I was about as prepared as I could've been to face life's challenges. However, I didn't face them well at all. In fact, I forgot everything I knew when I got hit square between the eyes with the realities of life.

What happened? At fourteen, I was raped. Where do you go with that?

What do you do with that? Well, I can only tell you what I did; and I can say with 100% certainty, I do not recommend it. Did I run to God for help like I had been taught? No! Did I run to my parents for help? No! I ran home and locked myself in my room. Alone. I locked the door behind me and locked everyone else out—including God.

I was scared.

Alone.

Angry.

Confused.

I was angry and confused because the God everyone told me I could trust, the God who was always watching over me, the God everyone told me would be there in my time of need, hadn't been. I felt God had let me down. You bet I was angry, and I demanded answers.

I cried out to this "God" and demanded he explain where I'd misunderstood. I didn't get answers, nor did I know where else to turn. I just knew I felt alone, scared, ashamed, out of control, and unloved.

If I wanted to be safe again, I had to take things into my own hands. The only way I knew to make sure no one could hurt me was to control every circumstance. That didn't seem hard in my little room. Only two ways in— the door or the window.

I sat with my back against the door and never took my eyes off the window. However, keeping myself safe that way obviously was not sustainable long term. I had to come out of my room at some point, and that meant developing much more elaborate attempts to keep myself safe. Constantly watching everything and everyone around me was exhausting work. I didn't have a choice if I wanted to be safe outside my room.

I didn't just want to feel safe, I wanted to be loved. I didn't believe I deserved it anymore, though, so that meant doing whatever it took to earn people's love. Doing *whatever it takes* when you are a teenage girl seeking love, as you can imagine, is not something you go around talking about, at least not in that generation.

So, I didn't talk about it. I didn't tell my friends, I didn't tell my parents, and I certainly didn't tell anyone at church. They have names for girls like that, you know. The isolation only led to more anger and more questions for which I demanded answers. More answers that never came. In hindsight, the most important question of all didn't come until recently.

The question was, "How can a loving God allow a faithful little girl to be destroyed in one night and then spend the next forty years allowing guilt and shame to destroy whatever had been left standing?" A better question is, "Why did I waste forty years of my life before I had the courage and strength to cry out, 'NO MORE?'"

Why was this the most important question? Because this question led to the truth.

The truth is, the victory over guilt and shame was already mine. The victory was mine the moment I accepted the sacrifice Jesus made on the cross for all my sins past, present, and future. The reality is, I chose to live in shame and disgrace by locking God out of my room and my life on that night. I chose not to live in the victorious life God had already planned and purposed for me before I was ever born. God had a plan to use what others had meant for evil in my life on that night for good in the lives of others—hence, this book.

The reality is, I chose to live in shame and disgrace by locking God out of my room and my life on that night. I chose not to live in the victorious life God had already planned and purposed for me before I was ever born.

That is my story. What about you? What brought you to this point? How did you, or your loved one, get here? Let's look at some other circumstances that can also lead to depression. Maybe one of them applies to you.

A circumstance in life that often causes people to fall into situational depression (depression resulting from a stressful situation in your life) is grief. I have experienced true grief twice in my life: once, at the age of twenty-six, when my older sister died; and again, decades later, when my father died suddenly just six months after my breakdown. We each deal with grief differently. There are even differences in how I dealt with these two tragic situations.

When my sister died, I was devastated, and it altered my life. It amplified what had already been started by the PTSD. I now suspect it was due, in large part, to my walk with God at the time.

Actually, it was my lack of a walk with God at the time that made the difference. I, once again, felt God had let me down. I cried out and demanded answers that, again, never came.

While I now understand horrible things do happen to good people, I also know God is in control. God allows bad things to happen. We choose whether to allow those bad things to change us for better or worse and in what ways they will alter our lives.

I said earlier my sister's death altered my life. That's not actually true. Circumstances, like my sister's death, have no physical power over me. If my life was altered, it's because I chose to alter it. Hard to admit, but true. My anger with God for letting me down, yet again, would not allow me to lean on the one source of strength I needed during that time of grief. Instead, I allowed my grief to control my thoughts and actions, not God. Therefore, I chose to walk through it alone.

God allows bad things to happen. We choose whether to allow those bad things to change us for better or worse and in what ways they will alter our lives.

Although I was equally devastated to lose my dad, the experience, the grief, was totally different. The circumstances were the same, but my response wasn't. Why? Because this time, I was walking with God. I was studying the Bible and spending time in prayer daily. I simply asked him to guide me through it. Most importantly, I believed he would.

I asked him to give me peace and comfort from my despair and wisdom to help my mother walk through her grief. I asked him to help me to continue to put one foot in front of the other until the days passed and grief's chokehold on my life released slightly.

As I waited for the grief to pass, I stepped away and prayed multiple times each day. I went into a quiet place, which in a house full of relatives was usually a bathroom, and I asked God to take my hand and lead me. I asked him to show his love to others through me. I asked him to use the funeral service to minister to those who might be attending who didn't know him like I did. Sometimes, I even asked him to help me breathe.

Why did I ask for such things, which by the world's standards are miniscule and unworthy of prayer time? I asked because I knew God cared about every detail of my life, no matter how small. I knew God loved me and wanted the best for me. God loves you too, and he wants to walk side by side with you no matter what challenges you currently face.

What if you're not experiencing PTSD or grief? What if you're struggling with one of these: codependency, loneliness, addictions, infertility, life-altering medical diagnosis, work stress, relationship stress, parenting stress, caregiver stress, attempts to keep up with the Joneses, handling life in the fast lane, or even personal choices you've made that haven't been the best? As a lifelong educator, I would be remiss after that long list if I didn't include "all of the above" as a choice.

These, and many others, are legitimate reasons to land in a state of depression. I know people, personally, who have experienced each of the issues listed above. I don't begin to understand the pain my friends have experienced. I also can't begin to imagine the pain you may be experiencing with whatever challenge you're facing. The only thing I know for certain is that circumstances don't matter.

> *Rainbows are the result of storms, butterflies are birthed after struggling to escape cocoons, glittery things come with high credit card bills, and green grass comes from high water bills, long weekend caretaking, and a lot of … fertilizer.*

Each of those circumstances is just a different road that leads to the same place—depression. Let me assure you, the depression you feel is real. The feelings of unworthiness, hopelessness, and helplessness are real; but the reason behind those feelings is not. Why? Because our thoughts are shaped by the belief that everything we see truly is what it appears to be. However, often, it's not.

An Honest Look at My Thoughts

We have all heard the sayings a million times: all that glitters is not gold,[3] or the grass is always greener.[4] The reality is, just because something looks good, doesn't mean it is. Good things often come after a struggle. Rainbows are the result of storms, butterflies are birthed after struggling to escape cocoons, glittery things come with high credit card bills, and green grass comes from high water bills, long weekends of caretaking, and a lot of … fertilizer.

While it may look like someone else is better off than you, you aren't seeing the entire picture. You're only looking at one, or sometimes two, small aspects of a complete life. You don't know what it cost that friend to have whatever it is you're admiring.

For instance, I know lots of people who have good jobs and nice houses. They own boats and take expensive vacations. They always wear the latest fashions and eat at the finest restaurants. Sometimes, I envy what they have, and I dream of having more money. For me, however, a look at the bigger picture reveals the truth.

Chapter 1

The truth is, happiness isn't always related to money. I've worked for the school system for almost thirty years, so most people's salaries are higher than mine. My husband drove a truck for FedEx. No big salary there either. We eat at inexpensive fast food restaurants, live in the least expensive home in the neighborhood. Our furniture is from a thrift store or garage sale, was handed down by friends and family, or we've had it since we got married. Did I mention we just celebrated thirty-five years of marriage?

I'm not by any means suggesting we are poor. Our bills are paid, and we have no credit card debt or car loans. We may live paycheck to paycheck, but we are rich indeed.

Although I may not have all the rich, glittery things my friends have, what I do have is certainly gold! I have a husband who loves and adores me, four healthy, happy, God-fearing, rule-following (for the most part) adult children, and eight equally blessed grandchildren.

> *The realization of how blessed and rich I truly am was the first step to acknowledging it wasn't my life that needed changing, it was my thinking.*

Okay, you're right; they're not perfect. I don't have a perfect husband, children, or grandchildren, and heaven knows I'm not a perfect wife or mother. Nevertheless, we have everything we need when we're together.

So, when I look at the bigger picture, my life seems pretty good just the way it is. All those fancy homes, cars, boats, vacations, or successful jobs don't seem as important anymore. Sure, I'd love to have it all, and some people do; however, I've discovered what truly makes me happy. Family. There's no amount of money you could pay me to give up what I have with my family.

The realization of how blessed and rich I truly am was the first step to acknowledging it wasn't my life that needed changing, it was my thinking. However, my thinking wasn't my only problem. I needed to examine the difference between what I believed to be true and what was really true.

An Honest Look at My Beliefs

The reason I felt helpless, hopeless, and unworthy was because I'd chosen, consciously or not, to believe the lies our enemy, the devil, was telling me rather than to trust in the truth of the Bible. I know that sounds crazy. No one who claims to know God would ever believe Satan's lies over God's truth. At least that's what I was thinking when someone first suggested that was my problem. I was wrong. I knew God, and yet I was still believing the enemy's lies.

In fact, Revelations 12:10 confirms the enemy continuously condemns us all. Let's look at a few of the lies to which I've fallen prey. Maybe you've been a victim as well.

The Lie	The Truth
I'm worthless	**I am God's masterpiece.** Ephesians 2:10 makes that clear. In Isaiah 43:4, God reminds me I'm of great value to him. I am precious to him, I am honored, and he loves me. It just overwhelms me to think the same God who created the universe created me. He created the powerful, majestic mountains and the clear, beautiful, peaceful sea. It's truly unfathomable to imagine that same powerful, peaceful God took the time to create me. John 3:16 says I have such great worth, God sent his only son to take my place on the cross; to save me from the consequences of my own sin. Now that is worthy!
I'm hopeless	**God has a wonderful plan for my life if I will only choose to follow it.** Psalm 139:16 explains God planned out my life before I was even born. He then created me to perfectly fit that plan. When things seem unbearable, it's easy to forget God's plan which, spoiler alert, ends with me spending eternity in heaven with him. That's reason enough to remain hopeful in my current situation. John 9:1-3 describes Jesus healing a blind man. When the people questioned why God made him blind at all, Jesus teaches a powerful lesson we often forget. Sometimes, things happen simply so the power of God can be seen by all. God is using my painful past for his glory. There's hope

The Lie	The Truth
I'm hopeless (cont.)	because my pain is not wasted. Romans 8:28 says God works all things out for good. This verse doesn't say for our current good, or for our comfort or convenience. It doesn't say we'll never have problems. We think in terms of our lifetime. God speaks in terms of eternity. We need to maintain that perspective when we see suffering. However, we can remain hopeful that uncomfortable, even downright painful, circumstances can be used to bring an understanding of him and his glory. If not for us, then for someone else. While it's difficult to see any good in the rape of a teenager, God is using my triumph over that pain to help give hope to others. My past pain is being used for others' eternal gain.
I'm not good enough	**I don't have to be enough – Jesus is enough!** The enemy got this one partially right. I'm not good enough. I never will be; which is why God sent Jesus. Jesus is enough. Romans 3:20-26 says he stands between God and me, so God doesn't see my sin; he sees Jesus and his payment for my sin on the cross.
I'm alone	**God is always with me. He will never leave me.** Deuteronomy 31:6 is just one of many places this promise is repeated in the Bible. I need to remember each time God issues this promise, he is speaking to one of his righteous servants. God walks with me when I'm walking with him. Philippians 1:6 assures us God will be faithful to stay with us so he can complete anything he has started in us. When we trust in him, he will be faithful to walk with us. We never walk alone.

Without the Truth, We Live in Defeat

Although I believe all these truths now, I lived in defeat for many years, allowing the lies from our enemy, Satan, to define my existence. I'm not the only one to fall prey to these lies. Exodus 2 describes how Moses lived in defeat for many years as well. After being Prince of Egypt and killing an Egyptian soldier he felt was mistreating the Israelites, Moses fled to the desert in fear.

Since we know God doesn't give us a spirit of fear (2 Timothy 1:7), we can be certain the fear Moses felt was Satan's attempt to get him off track. And it worked. Moses lived in the desert with his father-in-law for forty years tending his sheep, feeling unworthy and unable to help his people, the Israelites.

Years later, the Israelites themselves lived in defeat after their proud and victorious exit from slavery in Egypt. Satan began planting seeds of doubt in their minds as soon as the harsh reality of life in the desert set in. Rather than continue to trust the one true God whom they had just witnessed perform multiple signs, wonders, and miracles to free them from Egypt, they believed Satan's lies telling them life was better when they were slaves.

Because they lost faith, they spent forty years wandering in the desert rather than moving forward to claim the land God had promised them. God would continue to care for them. He would also allow them to walk alone until they were ready to trust him again.

I'm sure God was whispering gentle words of conviction to them because he still loved them and wanted them to return to him and his ways. Apparently, they weren't listening.

Just like Moses and the Israelites, I too lost faith in God. I also spent forty years believing the lies of the enemy designed to distract me from all the wonderful things God had planned for me. Because I believed in those lies, I wandered in the desert; not a literal one, of course, but a definite time of spiritual dryness in my life. I was convinced I was unworthy. I was unusable by God. I was lost!

I'm Not Lost; I'm Wandering

J. R. Tolkien believes "not all who wander are lost."[5] I believe he's right. While Moses felt lost in the desert tending sheep, God's original plan for

26

him to free the Israelites from slavery in Egypt didn't change. Moses may have been wandering, yet he was never lost. God knew right where he was taking Moses, and exactly when he would take him there.

The time spent wandering in the desert was simply a divine delay, a time of preparation, in order for Moses to fulfill God's purpose for him. Moses needed to learn to trust God and prepare for the calling God had on his life to free the Israelites.

Just like Moses, the Israelites felt lost as they spent forty years in the desert wandering in circles. God's plan to have the Israelites live victoriously in the promised land didn't change; it was just on hold until the Israelites were ready. According to God's plan, the victory belonged to both Moses and the Israelites from the beginning. The wandering came into play when they chose not to live in, or walk in, that victory.

> *Moses may have been wandering, yet he was never lost. God knew right where He was taking Moses, and exactly when he would take him there.*

I'm guilty, also. I chose not to live in victory for years. I felt lost! I felt alone, scared, and unworthy of doing anything of importance. However, as with Moses and the Israelites, God has had a plan for my life all along. In the same way as Moses and the Israelites, I needed a time of preparation during my journey through the desert.

Is it time to stop wandering? Is it time to leave the desert behind and live victoriously in the plan God has for your life? Only you can decide. As for me, it was well past time.

I needed to speak up about how I was hurting. I needed to quit pretending everything was fine, quit settling for life in the desert. I needed a lot of things; I just couldn't seem to open my mouth. I needed an intervention. I needed someone to step in and say, "Enough is enough. It's time to get help. You were made for so much more than this."

That intervention never came for me. My breakdown came first. But it can for you. I want to be that intervention for you. So, hear my heart when I say, "You've suffered long enough. It's time to get help. You were made for so much more than this!"

The Desire to Change

My life today is living proof we can overcome depression. We can walk in victory. There is hope. It's also proof that if we don't eliminate destructive habits, our destructive habits will eliminate us. Things will only change when we decide they need to change. Things will only get better when we decide to make them better.

> *If we don't eliminate destructive habits, our destructive habits will eliminate us. Things will only change when we decide they need to change. Things will only get better when we decide to make them better.*

For me, change came with the realization that it was no longer an option to continue to live the way I was. When my rubber band burst on that October day, I landed in a behavioral hospital, unable to even care for myself. Something had to change. It wasn't a choice. I wanted to live. I wanted to survive. No, that's not even true. I had been surviving for forty years. I wanted to thrive.

To do that, however, I had to be willing to struggle through the hard work it was going to take to deal with the issue I'd been burying for forty years. I had to be willing to do the hard work necessary to change the way I looked at my past, my present, and my future. I had to re-examine my beliefs, my thoughts, and my habits. Nothing was sacred. If it wasn't productive, it had to go. The process wasn't easy; still, I can say with 100% certainty it was worth it.

Inspiration Suggestions

➢ *Others were given in exchange for you. I traded their lives for yours because you are precious to me. You are honored, and I love you. Isaiah 43:4*

➢ *You intended to harm me, but God intended it all for good. He brought me to this position, so I could save the lives of many people. Genesis 50:20*

➢ *This happened so the power of God could be seen in him. John 9:3b*

> ➤ *So be strong and courageous! Do not be afraid and do not panic before them. For the Lord your God will personally go ahead of you. He will neither fail you nor abandon you. Deuteronomy 31:6*

> ➤ *You have allowed me to suffer much hardship, but you will restore me to life again and lift me up from the depths of the earth. Psalm 71:20*

> ➤ *If you don't like where you are, move. You're not a tree. Jim Rohn*

> ➤ *Yesterday is not ours to recover, but tomorrow is ours to win or lose. Lyndon B. Johnson*

> ➤ *We must all suffer from one of two pains: the pain of discipline or the pain of regret. The difference is discipline weighs ounces while regret weighs tons. Jim Rohn*

> ➤ *We are never defeated unless we give up on God. Ronald Reagan*

Reflect

1. Are you ready to stop simply surviving and learn how to truly live, even if it requires some hard work?

2. What is testing the tensile strength of your emotions right now? Are you ready to break?

3. How did you get here? Did something specific happen, or has the weight of the world just built up over time?

4. How strong is your faith background? Is it strong enough to withstand a crisis?

5. Do you run to God or blame him when life hits you between the eyes?

6. Do you feel worthless, hopeless, helpless, or unlovable? Which of the enemy's lies are behind those feelings?

7. Have you wandered off course with God's plan for your life and gotten distracted?

8. What area of your heart does God need to heal?

9. What destructive habits do you need to change?

10. Which Inspiration Suggestions did you choose to explore, and which stood out that you'd like to remember?

11. What action steps do you need to take to implement what you've discovered in this chapter?

2

I (Don't) Need Everyone to Like Me

Approval Addiction & People Pleasing

I don't measure up?
I didn't make the team?
You didn't like my meatloaf?
Every day we let others decide whether we're good enough. While that can be a bad thing, sometimes it's valid to have an assessment or standard we must meet. I don't want a doctor operating on me who hasn't successfully finished medical school. However, losing sleep because someone doesn't like my meatloaf is taking it a little too far. That's exactly where I found myself.

Living Life on a Stage

We're constantly being compared and judged against some standard set up by someone else. When I was in school, I focused on getting the best grades, earning first chair in band, or winning first place in gymnastics.

At home, I tried to clean my plate, keep my room neat, and be in bed on time. As a young adult, the focus changed. I needed to be the best at job interviews, get top marks on performance appraisals, and later be the best wife and mother.

Now, as a wife of thirty-five years, mother of four adult children, grandmother to five grandsons and three granddaughters, as well as being an educational administrator, I realize the need to be the best never stops.

Constantly trying to be the best was a never-ending cycle. I essentially lived every moment of my life on a stage—always seeking someone's applause. I always wanted someone to catch me being good, to notice I was good at something. However, the Bible warns against the need to be seen.

I was only worthy when I made someone happy 100% of the time. At 99%, I became a failure. I became unworthy.

In Matthew 6:1, Jesus tells us, "Watch out! Don't do your good deeds publicly, to be admired by others, for you will lose the reward from your Father in heaven." That's pretty straightforward. We can enjoy the praises of men now or the praises of God forever.

Another reminder comes in Matthew 23:5-7, "Everything they do is for show… they love to sit at the head table at banquets and in the seats of honor in the synagogues. They love to receive respectful greetings as they walk in the marketplaces, and to be called 'Rabbi.'" In other words, they constantly called attention to themselves. They wanted to be recognized and honored for their accomplishments. Yep, that was me.

I always wanted to be in the front row or have the best role or the… whatever. At some point, I'm not exactly sure when, I realized the truth: applause and recognition from others is temporary.

No one in my life today knows or cares whether I made the honor roll, was a cheerleader, or received Employee of the Month and Teacher of the Year honors. Yet, those are all achievements I worked incredibly hard to earn. They're all achievements I thought would make me *somebody*. However, I still felt like nobody. Why was it so important to me to be *somebody* in the first place? Why did I need them to approve of me?

It all goes back to that scared, hurt fourteen-year-old girl who decided she was unworthy of love or respect. It became my life's mission to be worthy. I became completely focused on not only doing everything right but being seen doing it right. In my mind, I was only worthy when I made someone happy 100% of the time. At 99%, I became a failure. I became unworthy.

Obviously, this was an extremely distorted view, yet it was my reality at that time. It was the beginning of decades of attention-seeking behaviors that were not only unproductive but destructive, because I sought to please others no matter what it cost me.

The biggest cost was my self-esteem. I felt worthless. My needs and wants didn't matter. I thought my only value was in pleasing others. I was like a crack addict living for that next fix, only my fix was someone's words of praise. For so many years, I just wanted to be somebody important. Somebody others would look up to and respect.

It wasn't until I had my breakdown that I realized that, even though I had always wanted to be somebody, in reality, I already was.

I was somebody because God made me somebody. He loved everything about me and thought I had incredible value. After all, he made me. And that value couldn't be taken away from me by what was done to me. With that reality in mind, I had to re-examine why I'd spent so much time worrying about what others thought.

Why Do We Care What Others Think?

God created the need within us to feel loved. His intention was to have that longing draw us closer to him. The problem is, we fill this need with human love and adoration rather than God's.

For instance, as my husband would plan date nights, he would ask me what I wanted to do. I remember thinking, "Just make me feel special." I wanted to know I mattered. I needed to know I was worthy of love.

My husband certainly thought I was worthy of love. However, he was also human. No matter how hard he tried, he couldn't read my mind. He had no idea what would make me feel special. Sometimes the restaurant he picked wasn't my favorite or the romantic vacation didn't live up to my expectations. It all reminded me of that first meatloaf I made him that didn't measure up.

Apparently, his mom and mine cooked meatloaf in completely different ways. The meatloaf from my childhood, and the comfort it brought me, just didn't match the meatloaf he remembered. That's when I started losing sleep over his dislike of my meatloaf. Silly, right?

What I didn't realize during those sleepless nights is that, while I felt like a failure when he didn't like my meatloaf, that wasn't my husband's fault. He isn't responsible for my self-esteem. It's his job to love me, and he truly does.

His approval or disapproval doesn't change my value. Except in my mind.

I'm valuable because I'm the daughter of the King of Kings. My husband's inability to make me feel special didn't make me any less special. I'm special because God says I'm special, I'm honored, and he loves me (Isaiah 43:4). Unfortunately, sometimes I still forget who I am and go to great lengths to gain my husband's approval and feel loved.

While my husband's approval might rightfully affect decisions I make because we share a household and a life together, what about the approval of friends? How should they affect me or the decisions I make? A better question might be: should the approval of my friends affect me or the decisions I make?

> *The approval or disapproval of others doesn't change my value. Except in my mind.*

Just as with my husband, there may be a legitimate reason I want the approval of close friends. What about friends I haven't seen for years? Many would argue if we don't see someone anymore, we certainly aren't trying to please or impress them.

I don't believe that. The hurtful words of schoolyard bullies and the rejection we feel when we're excluded from popular social circles can continue to impact our lives decades later. We may still be trying to please or impress people who've long since been out of our lives, even if we do it subconsciously.

The problem with allowing these earlier relationships to affect us is that we are giving up control of our current life to hurtful words and actions from our past.

At a particularly dark time, as I struggled with those hurtful words and actions, someone told me a story about refusing to allow our past to control our present. The story tells of a woman who was celebrating her 100th birthday. She'd been attacked as a young woman, and her attacker had left her badly beaten, crippled, and blind.

A reporter conducting an interview for her birthday celebration asked, "How can you live with what that man did to you?" She answered, "I gave that man one night of my life. He'll never have another moment, as long as I live!"

What a powerful statement. *She* had the power to control how she felt about herself and her future, not the man who hurt her so many years before. The defining moment so many people remembered and used as a filter through which to see her didn't matter to her. For her, that night was just one event among millions of others she'd experienced throughout her life. No more, no less. It held no power over her.

I wanted to be just like that woman. I didn't want my past to have power over me. However, at the time I heard her story, it did. I had handed over control of my life to my past and didn't know how to take it back.

She had the power to control how she felt about herself and her future, not the man who hurt her so many years before.

As Whitney Houston points out in her song "Greatest Love of All," people can hurt me and take things from me. Unfortunately, I can't always stop them from hurting me physically. What I can do is stop them from hurting me emotionally. That's the one thing they can't take from me—my feelings about myself. My self-respect.

I can give it away, though. And I did. I lost respect for myself. I judged myself based on the actions of a few and what I believed others would think of me because of that. And there it is again. I was worrying about what others thought of me.

In the end, what others think and whether they love and respect me isn't important. What I think of me is more important than what anyone else thinks of me. The power to prevent the words and actions of others from hurting or controlling me comes when I learn to love and respect myself. When I learn to love myself, the thoughts of those around me become insignificant.

Life is NOT Pay for Performance

While we don't have to please friends, neighbors, or acquaintances from our past, we often need to please an employer. Unless we're independently wealthy, that is.

Many employers these days use a pay-for-performance or merit-based system of evaluation. These types of systems require us to earn points to get to a higher rating, to prove our worth to someone we think matters. We have to do more in order to get more.

The problem comes when we apply this employment evaluation system to our lives. I often make that mistake and feel like my reward for performance in life is given out the same way. I feel like I'm always working towards that next evaluation, whether it be annually, monthly, weekly, hourly, or—worse yet—by the item or action.

I learned about this conditional evaluation of my worth as a child. My dad used to tell my sisters and me he would pay us five cents for every dandelion we could pull out of the yard; however, only if we got the root.

Analysis: Root = worthy. No root = unworthy. I worked tirelessly to make sure I got the root, even if it meant fewer dandelions, because I needed to feel worthy. I wanted to please my daddy.

When I grew older, I worked for a large corporation where I often heard people who'd just made a mistake say, "One *whoops* wipes out 100 *atta boys*." They were essentially saying we're only as valuable as our last accomplishment. I said whoops a lot, so once again I found myself working to please people.

Even in my current position with the local school system, everything I do is evaluated based on a pay-for-performance model. If I show all the right people I can do all the right things, check all the right boxes, and never make any public mistakes, then, and only then, can I receive the coveted "highly effective" rating.

Do you know how few people actually meet that standard? I can assure you it's a small percentage. Everyone else is "effective." Nobody wants to be merely "effective." Accurate or not, we all consider ourselves "highly effective."

I've learned the approval of men is nothing compared to the approval of God.

However, no matter how hard I try, I'll never truly measure up to that "highly effective" rating. I might receive it on an evaluation because a supervisor deems me worthy of the higher rating, yet I'll never be able to truly check all those boxes.

In the meantime, while I was killing myself trying, I felt overwhelmingly unworthy. No matter how much I did, or how well I did it, I could never measure up. Yet again, my life was summed up by trying to meet someone else's standard, to please other people.

I look back now and realize none of that really matters. Nor do the opinions of those I've tried so hard to please. I've learned the approval of men is nothing compared to the approval of God.

In Galatians 1:10 Paul asks, "Am I trying to win human approval? No indeed! What I want is God's approval! Am I trying to be popular with people? If I were still trying to do so, I would not be a servant of Christ." (GNT)

I want to be a servant of Christ; therefore, it's time to stop seeking human approval. I want to seek after God's approval, which he freely gives me when I live for his glory and not my own.

One word of caution, though. I wouldn't go tell your boss you don't care what he thinks anymore; at least not if you want to keep your job. While we can seek after God's approval more than man's, we still live in a world where our paycheck comes from meeting standards set out by our employer.

A friend summed it up well when he said, "I work to a standard, not to a clock." If we do all things with integrity, to please God and to meet his standard, our worldly evaluation should fall into place. When I work to please God, to meet his standard of honesty, integrity, and love for others, I will be "highly effective."

What Really Matters?

Husbands, friends, neighbors, coworkers, and bosses are all important, of course. Keeping them relatively happy makes life during our short time on this earth a little easier. However, not when we constantly sacrifice our own wants and needs to make them happy.

Besides, what matters is not whether others are happy with us. What matters is whether God is happy with us. What matters most, though, is whether we'll spend eternity in heaven in a constant state of worship and fellowship with God. I can't begin to imagine what that'll be like. The closest I've come is a recent Beth Moore Conference.

Although it was an incredibly powerful experience, it was only a glimpse of the powerful joy we'll feel in heaven. The temporary joy I might experience when someone catches me doing something good can't compare to the joy of heaven. Matthew 16:26 reminds us it means nothing to "conquer the world" if we forget who we are in Christ.

In other words, it means nothing to be somebody without Jesus. Nothing on this earth is as valuable as the abundant life we receive not only in heaven, but right now through the Holy Spirit living within us.

I have to choose each day what's important. I have to decide what I'll focus on each minute of each day. Will it be the glory and praise of those around me and the worldly success that could be gone in an instant or the abundant life that brings freedom from performance pressure in this world right now and forever? As for me, I choose to serve God! (Joshua 24:15)

What about you? Will you choose to spend your time, energy, and emotion on receiving the abundant life he offers rather than living in the performance trap set by the world?

Inspiration Suggestions

➢ *People pleasing is no longer an option because I am adopting the radical belief that my ideas, thoughts, and opinions matter too. Unknown*

➢ *If you live for people's acceptance, you will die from their rejection. Lecrae*

➢ *If you are an approval addict, your behavior is as easy to control as that of any other junkie. All a manipulator need do is a simple two-step process: Give you what you crave, and then threaten to take it away. Every drug dealer in the world plays this game. Harriet B. Braiker*

➢ *Suppose you could gain everything in the whole world and lost your soul. Was it worth it? Billy Graham*

➢ *Like any addict, insecure people look for a "fix" when they get shaky. They need someone to reaffirm them and assure them everything is all right and they are acceptable. When a person has an addiction, the things they are addicted to are on their mind most of the time. Therefore, if a person is an approval addict, he or she will have an abnormal concern and an abundance of thoughts about what people think of them. Joyce Meyer*

➢ *Song – "He Knows My Name" by Francesca Battistelli**

➢ *Song – "Great Are You Lord" by All Sons & Daughters**

➢ *Song – "More Beautiful You" by Jonny Diaz**

> ➤ *Song – "Who I Am" by Blanca**

*Video available at https://bit.ly/2I38TXv

Reflect

1. Who from your past are you still trying to please or impress?

2. What hurtful words or actions from your past have stolen your ability to love and respect yourself?

3. What steps do you need to take to love and respect yourself again?

4. In what ways do you seek out the attention of others for validation of your worthiness or lovability?

5. What changes do you need to make to start living to God's standard?

6. Are you caught in the performance trap of this world? What can you do to start focusing on pleasing God over man?

7. What areas of your heart does God need to heal?

8. What destructive habits do you need to change?

9. Which Inspiration Suggestions did you choose to explore, and which stood out you'd like to remember?

10. What action steps do you need to take to implement what you've discovered in this chapter?

3

I (Don't) Need to Do Everything Right

Perfectionism

Everyone makes mistakes! That's what they tell me anyway. If that's true, why do I feel like I'm the only one ever making them? Even if others do make mistakes, my mistakes seem to be the only ones anyone sees. However, there's a distinct difference between failing in the eyes of man and failing in the eyes of God.

No One Is Perfect

Failing in the eyes of man means I didn't live up to the expectations of another human. I can keep trying, and if I work hard enough, I might eventually meet their standard. It's possible to get a perfect score when I'm trying to meet the standards of men. A perfect score from an imperfect human; now that's an interesting concept.

Why do I say they're imperfect humans? Although we can get a perfect score on their assessment, we're not perfect. Neither are they. Ecclesiastes 7:20 says, "Not a single person on earth is always good and never sins." This concept is reinforced in Romans 3:10, which says, "No one is righteous – not even one."

If these scriptures are true, why do I constantly feel the need to be perfect or feel like a failure when things don't go the way they should? Nobody else seems to worry about it; so why do I? I tend to tell others "it's no big deal" when they do something wrong; however, I never give myself that same break. It's always a big deal when I do something wrong. Could it be I expect too much of myself? I only see the bad in myself and only the good in others.

There's a term for this malady, which means I'm not the only one who feels this way. It's called self-hatred. I believe everything I do is wrong or doesn't measure up. In reality, that's true. I'll never measure up to the perfect standard of Jesus. However, neither will anyone else. Remember, no one is righteous; not even one. (Romans 3:10)

I suspect the solution starts with seeing myself the way God sees me, which means lowering my expectations of myself. After all, I'm human. I will make mistakes. Yet, God loves me just the way I am.

I see myself as an imperfect human. God sees me as a perfectly flawed human. What I mean is, he made me exactly the way I am. I meet his design plan perfectly.

In the story of the adulteress woman, Jesus told the crowd only those who had never sinned could judge her. (John 8:8) Why is that? After all, she'd been caught red-handed breaking the law. She was guilty. That fact was not up for debate.

Jesus did this to point out none of them were innocent of sin either. God catches every one of us red-handed breaking his law at some point. Jesus knew none of those people were perfect; none of them could say they'd never done anything wrong. They were all guilty in God's eyes.

The same is still true. None of us are perfect. We've all done something we hope no one ever sees or hears about.

I think the lesson Jesus was trying to teach us is about our role in the sins of other people. More precisely, the lack of a role for us in the sins of other people. It's not our job to judge sin. Only the righteous can judge sin, and only God is righteous. Therefore, only God has the right to judge me or anyone else.

Avoid Comparisons

Once we realize we aren't righteous, and we're no better or worse than all the other sinners around us, it's time to realize we don't need to compete with anyone else. It's not a matter of who has less sin, who is "holier than thou," because the question of sin is not measured in degrees. It's a yes or no question.

If we have to compare ourselves with someone, Jesus is the only option. He's the only one without sin. In 2 Corinthians 10:12, we're told it's not wise to compare ourselves against others. It's not a competition, or at least not with each other. The standard we should be striving to reach is Christ, not someone else.

It's not a matter of who wins and who loses. It's like the Olympics. There's only one winner. Essentially, everyone else is a loser if you want to look at it that way. In fact, I've heard it's psychologically better to win the bronze medal than the silver.

It's not a matter of who has less sin; who is "holier than thou," because the question of sin is not measured in degrees. It's a yes or no question.

I had to think about that one for a while before I finally figured out why. Although they're both, by definition, losers, the bronze medalist often feels like a winner, while the silver medalist feels like a loser. Think about it. I'll give you a hint. It's about their emotional well-being.

The bronze medalist is ecstatic to even make it to the medal stand. She just barely squeaked by the others to get that recognition. She's grateful to even be there.

On the other hand, the silver medalist will always feel like she just barely missed reaching her dream. She fell just short of victory. She came so close to getting the recognition she deserved. She'll always wonder *what if*. What if she'd done this, or that, differently? She came so close. Surely there was something she could've done to win.

The reality is, they both fell short. Every competitor fell short except the winner. In life, we all fall short. In our case, we'll never be the winner no matter how hard we try. Why?

Because, in our case, the winner is Christ. He's our measuring stick and by that measure the rest of us are all equal. And all failures. I know we're not better than others, and I get that part; however, we're not worse either. That's the part I still have trouble believing. We may sin differently, yet we all sin.

So now that you're feeling a little self-hatred too, what should you do? Just like me, it's time to quit trying to be what others think you should be, or who you think you should be, and just be who God made you to be.

Get Back Up

Now that we recognize the existence of sin in our lives, the question is what are we going to do about it? Proverbs 24:16 reminds us the godly may trip, but they will get up again.

I can certainly attest to that fact. I've fallen multiple times in my life. I'm not especially proud to admit it, but some of those times I fell down and stayed down. Yep, I've wallowed in the deep, dark pit of self-pity. I'm not alone, though. Everyone falls. Everyone has lived in the pit at one time or another. It's normal. But when we fall, God wants us to get back up and live victoriously.

A little boy in the poem *The Race* teaches us the importance of getting back up.[1] He's encouraged to fight through his failures by the thought of his father waiting at the finish line for him. I need to follow his example. I also need to stop beating myself up when I stumble and fall.

> *It's not about me. I'm not righteous. It's about Jesus, who is righteous and submits his work on my behalf.*

Finally, I need to accept my mistakes, learn from them, and keep moving in the direction of the finish line. I need to let go of what's gone wrong and finish my race. If I do what's right to the best of my ability, even when I fall, God, my heavenly father, will be waiting at the finish line. He's waiting to greet me with love whether I finish first or last.

How do I know for sure God will be waiting for me? How do I know he'll be happy to see me? It goes back to seeing myself through God's eyes. I find it hard to overlook all my mistakes and the times I pushed him away. It's hard to keep going when that finish line is so far away, and I already feel like I've failed. God doesn't see me that way, though.

God doesn't see all the times I've wanted to quit because it just seemed hopeless. God sees the one time I got back up and tried again anyway. More importantly, God sees the work Jesus did on the cross on my behalf.

So how do I quit focusing on all I've done wrong and start focusing on all Jesus has done right? By remembering it's not about me. I'm not righteous. It's about Jesus, who is righteous and submits his work on my behalf.

Say what? From the perspective of a lifelong educator, that certainly sounds like cheating. How can that be allowed?

Not only is it allowed, with God, it's the only way.

Jesus stands between God and me. God only sees me through the cleansing blood of the sacrifice on the cross Jesus made on my behalf. I know that—in my head. However, there's always that little voice that reminds me of my past. It reminds me of all that I've done wrong.

Condemnation or Conviction

That little voice is our enemy, Satan. Condemnation, a focus on all I do wrong, is not from God. Revelations 12:10 tells us Satan continuously condemns us.

Every time Satan tries to condemn me, I have the power to choose whether to believe him.

He's very quick to point out all my mistakes and incessantly reminds me of them. He points out my problems then convinces me there's no answer, no solution, no way out of the mess I've made of my life. He convinces me this one mistake, no matter how small, is enough to ruin my life forever. This one little bad decision is the proverbial straw.

He tries to convince me the accumulation of failure in my life is now more than God can forgive. The scales have tipped too far. I can't recover.

However, if I know that's not true, if I know the truth that Jesus died on the cross to save me from my sins, why do I believe him? If you've ever heard these little whisperings of condemnation, you know exactly why. The enemy can be very convincing.

It's simple. All he has to do is create doubt. Doubt makes me question what I believe and what I know to be true. Remember how easily he confused Eve? All he did was make her doubt what God told her was true.

For many years I believed the lies. I allowed myself to doubt God's promises to me. All right, I confess; sometimes I still do. The good news is, every time Satan tries to condemn me, I have the power to choose whether to believe him.

Although it may seem like he has power over my mind, he doesn't. He has no power that I, personally, haven't given him.

I can choose whether to allow the seeds of doubt to grow or to trust God's Word and his promises. Now that I know what Satan's up to, I can choose not to believe his condemnation. I can choose not to feel like a failure.

Instead, I can choose to allow God's conviction to show me the answer to my problems and remind me through Jesus there's always hope.

Conviction is different than condemnation. Conviction is from God. It's a simple, gentle nudge that encourages me to change my behavior so I can restore my relationship with him.

It doesn't show me my problem, like condemnation; it shows me the answer to my problem—Jesus.

Let's think in terms of a relationship we might better understand, marriage. When I do something that hurts my husband's feelings, he doesn't suddenly stop loving me. He still loves me. He still wants to spend the rest of his life with me. However, at that moment, he's disappointed in my thoughtless, inconsiderate behavior.

My actions have caused tension in our relationship. His gentle reminder I've hurt him will create a desire within me to make things right, a desire to restore our relationship.

Conviction is just like that. God whispers to me, "I'm disappointed in that choice, or that action. I want us to be close again. I miss our closeness. I miss you. Please come back. I want you in my life."

Romans 2:4 says, "Godly sorrow leads to repentance." What's repentance? What does God want me to see and to do when I hear his gentle words?

Conviction is different than condemnation. Conviction is from God. It's a simple, gentle nudge that encourages me to change my behavior so I can restore my relationship with him.

Repentance means I allow God's conviction to point me to the sacrifice of Jesus on the cross. The death of Christ on the cross for my sins is the only way to restore my relationship with God. Why is that?

Romans 6:23 tells us why. It says, "The wages of sin is death, but the free gift of God is eternal life through Christ Jesus our Lord."

When I repent, I agree with God my actions weren't in line with his will for my life. Basically, I agree with God I've sinned. When I agree I've sinned, I must also agree to accept the punishment for sin, which is spiritual death—an eternity separated from God.

Let me say that again so it can sink in. When I agree I have sinned, I acknowledge I deserve to spend eternity away from God. In Hell.

If I want to spend eternity with God, which I definitely do, I have a need for someone else to pay that wage—spiritual death—for me. Therefore, the payment by Jesus for my sins on that cross is the only solution to my problem.

The moment I acknowledge that fact, just like the thief on the cross, I too will live with Christ in paradise for eternity (Luke 23:39-43).

That's great news. My eternity is secure with God! What about now, though? What about today? Each time I sin, it creates a distance in my relationship with God. I must continually listen to his guidance, his conviction, reminding me something is not right in our relationship. There's tension.

He not only wants me to finish my race strong, so I can spend eternity with him, he also wants to enjoy the journey with me now along the way. He wants to run right beside me and encourage me when I stumble. He wants to pick me up when I fall; and when I can't run any further, he wants to carry me. He wants to do it with me not just for me.

I don't know about you, but the choice between guilt and grace, condemnation and conviction, is very clear to me now. I choose conviction. I choose the opportunity of an eternity in heaven Jesus died to give me. I choose to accept I'm not perfect.

I want to recognize and repent from the mess I've made of my life and do what I need to do to restore my relationship with God. I want to run the race with him, not on my own.

What about you? Will you choose condemnation, doubt, and defeat? Or will you choose conviction, correction, and restoration?

I'm not perfect. I fail in the eyes of man every single day in some way or another. I'll never be perfect in their eyes. I also fail in the eyes of God every single day. However, because I allow God's conviction and take the necessary steps to restore our relationship, I can enjoy the journey with him now and still look forward to the day I get to heaven and hear him say, "Well done my good and faithful servant." (Matthew 25:23)

Inspiration Suggestions

➢ *I have never known anyone to accept Christ's redemption and later regret it. Billy Graham*

➢ *Perfectionism is just an excuse for self-criticism. Sharon Martin*

> ➢ *Perfectionism is self-abuse of the highest order. Anne Wilson Schaef*

> ➢ *I might not be perfect, but neither are you. So, go and check your mistakes before rating mine. Unknown*

> ➢ *Song – "Grace Wins" by Matthew West*

> ➢ *Song – "I Have Decided" by Elevation Worship**

> ➢ *Song – "Free to Be Me" by Francesca Battistelli**

> ➢ *Song – "Broken Things" by Matthew West**

> ➢ *Song – "O Come to the Altar" by Elevation Worship**

Video available at https://bit.ly/2I38TXv

Reflect

1. In what ways have you failed to meet the standards of men recently?

2. In what ways have you failed to meet the standards of God recently?

3. In what ways do you compare yourself to others? Why do you feel the need to compare at all?

4. What words of condemnation has Satan whispered to you recently? Do you believe them?

5. How could you tell it was condemnation rather than conviction?

6. What can you do to overcome condemnation's power over you?

7. Has God convicted you about something recently? How could you tell it was conviction and not condemnation?

8. If you felt convicted about something, did you repent and receive God's forgiveness? How did that make you feel?

9. Have you accepted the sacrifice Christ made on the cross to pay the price for your sins? If not, what's holding you back?

10. Which Inspiration Suggestions did you choose to explore, and which stood out you'd like to remember?

11. What action steps do you need to take to implement what you've discovered in this chapter?

NOTE: If you're not sure how to accept the sacrifice Christ made on the cross to pay the price for your sins, see the Steps to Salvation on the next page.

For questions or prayer about this decision, see what Billy Graham has to say at https://peacewithgod.net/ or contact me personally at vicki@sadnesstojoy.com.

Steps to Salvation

- ***Understand the depth of God's love for you*** *– For God so loved the world that he gave his one and only Son, that whoever believes in him shall not perish but have eternal life. John 3:16 (NIV)*

- ***Admit you are a sinner*** *– No one is righteous; not even one. Romans 3:10*

- ***Understand the price for sin is spiritual death*** *– For the wages of sin is death, but the free gift of God is eternal life through Christ Jesus our Lord. Romans 6:23*

- ***Realize Jesus paid the price for your sin*** *– But God showed his great love for us by sending Christ to die for us while we were still sinners. Romans 5:8*

- ***Believe Jesus defeated death & declare him as Lord*** *– If you declare with your mouth, "Jesus is Lord," and believe in your heart that God raised him from the dead, you will be saved. For it is with your heart that you believe and are justified, and it is with your mouth that you profess your faith and are saved. Romans 10:9-10*

4

I (Don't) Need to Be in Control

Control Freak

When control is jerked from you, and bad things happen, you can't help but think things could have been different, could have been better, if you had just been in control. If I'm in control, no one can hurt me! Really? Then how come every time things don't go the way I planned, I end up an emotional wreck, feeling like a failure in life?

What about those times I was in control? I planned everything out perfectly; and yet, something went wrong. Someone wasn't happy. Something didn't work out just right. It rained! Although none of these things can hurt me physically, they can hurt me emotionally—if I let them.

When I Think I'm In Control – I'm Really Not

After you've experienced an out-of-control moment with such devastating consequences, as I did, you begin to believe being in control equals safety. Nobody can hurt me if I can just control everything. After forty years of trying, I can assure you, you can NOT control everything.

Let's talk about control and theme parks. A family outing took us to Silver Dollar City in Branson, Missouri, near my parents' home in Springfield. You can guess how it goes with a control freak when planning a day at a theme park. When you spend that much money for tickets, meals, snacks, and souvenirs, you want everything to be picture-postcard perfect. I packed extra patience for the lines, which is always necessary when you ride Fire in the Hole, a local favorite. It has managed to hold its own as newer, faster thrill rides have moved into town.

When it rains, literally or figuratively, I have two choices. I can sit inside and pout about all the things I can't do; or I can put up my umbrella and enjoy all the things I can do.

I saw the clouds rolling in as we stood in the seemingly never-ending line, going around and around through the maze of ropes corralling everyone in the same direction.

Fire in the Hole is an indoor roller coaster staged in an old mine. The last portion of the wait is spent inside the entrance to the mine, where we were out of sight of those threatening clouds.

After what seemed like a minute and a half on the actual coaster, we emerged from the mine tunnel exit to, you guessed it, rain. This was not just a spring shower. It was a storm of biblical proportions complete with deafening thunder and frequent blinding lightning.

All right, I lied. We didn't actually emerge from the tunnel. We huddled in that tunnel as I felt all my planning go down the tubes. The one thing I hadn't planned for was rain. As far as I was concerned, our day was completely ruined, and we might as well go home. And it wasn't even 10:00 am! No matter how hard I try, I can't control the rain.

As I've grown older, and spent hours in therapy, I've come to understand better what I learned that day. I can't control everything. In fact, I can't control most things. As my therapist continuously reminds me, I can't control people, places, things, or events.

When it rains, literally or figuratively, I have two choices. I can sit inside and pout about all the things I can't do, or I can put up my umbrella and enjoy all the things I can do.

My dad tried to teach me that lesson on that rainy day at Silver Dollar City. He made jokes and kept things light-hearted until the storm slowed down enough for us to run across the path to the gift shop. We all got ponchos and went about enjoying the rest of our day—happily, I might add.

Sometimes I Fail to Step Out, Even When I'm Called

When I try to live in control of everything, sometimes I fail to take risks. It hurts when I think about all the opportunities for joy I missed because of little things I couldn't control. I was afraid to try. Matthew 14:22-33 tells us of someone else who almost made that same mistake.

Peter stood in the boat in the middle of the stormy sea. Jesus walked out on the water and beckoned Peter to step out of the boat and walk out on the water to him. To get out of that boat took amazing courage and faith. It took more faith than I could've mustered. Peter could no more control those overwhelming waves than I could control the rain.

If Peter had been a control freak, he would've told Jesus to wait until the storm had stopped. Or better yet, bring the boat safely to the shore and meet Peter there. I truly believe Peter wanted to trust God had a plan for this moment in his life. He desperately wanted to believe God had all the details under control, especially those huge, terrifying waves.

With that trust in mind, Peter eventually talked himself into believing that Jesus wouldn't ask him to do something he couldn't physically do; he stepped out on the choppy water and took that first step. Rather than be awed by the impossible fact he was walking on water, he instead heard those little whispers of doubt and defeat. That's all it took. Satan spoke a few words of doubt, and it was over.

Peter's focus was no longer on Jesus and the plan to bring him safely out on the water to him. Peter's focus promptly went to the voice of doubt, the voice telling him that people don't walk on water!

When Peter started to focus on whether he could actually walk on the water under his own power, he started to sink. Although terrified as he started to flounder in the tumultuous waves, Peter at least was smart enough to cry out for help rather than crawl back in the boat and hide.

This time, he chose to focus on the voice of truth. Peter chose to give up personal control, allow God to take him where he wanted him to go, and trust he would get there safely despite what appeared to be overwhelming odds.

Giving up control is not something with which I'm personally comfortable. Actually, that's an extreme exaggeration! It's not a concept with which I'm even remotely familiar. Peter was obviously much stronger in his faith amidst crisis than I am in mine. If I couldn't control those waves, I not only wouldn't have been able to get out of the boat to walk on water, I probably would never have been able to even leave the shore. However, when I'm not willing to get out of the boat, I can't enjoy the opportunity of walking with God.

After my sister died, leaving three small children without a mother, my willingness to take risks greatly diminished. I remember when my kids were younger, they always wanted me to go on roller coasters with them. You know the ones I'm talking about—the ones with an almost vertical drop or barrel rolls where you feel like you're going to fly out of the car and smash to the concrete far below. Don't forget the dueling coasters where the two cars on different tracks go past each other so closely you literally feel like you can reach out and high-five the person racing past you.

Although I did go on them occasionally, I was so overwhelmingly terrified I could hardly breathe. Was I simply afraid of death? No. I was terrified of leaving my children without a mother. That one thought caused me to miss out on sharing many amazing experiences with my children. When I fail to step out, I miss out.

Sometimes I Step Out, Even When I'm Not Called

I miss out on things when I don't step out to meet Jesus on the water. What happens when I step out to do things and Jesus isn't out there calling me to him? I've lost many hours of sleep over stepping out to do things God clearly hasn't called me to do.

For as long as I can remember, I've felt the need to fix things. I'm a problem solver. In fact, it's my number one strength on the StrengthsFinder assessment.[1] I've always felt the need to save people from suffering from the circumstances in their lives. I hurt, and I didn't want anyone else to hurt.

It makes sense, but it's not how things work. Remember, I can't control people, places, things, or events. That simple fact escaped me for many years as I continuously tried to fix (control) people and what I perceived as problems.

Because I spent my life filled with a need to control everything in order to be happy, I often felt responsible for the happiness of others. I wanted to keep them safe from the pain I'd experienced. I wanted to save them from the consequences of their actions, which I could clearly see only because I'd already suffered them. I suppose this feeling of responsibility for others started when I began getting help for my years of hurting.

As I dealt with my pain and heartache, I made a commitment to do everything I could to save others from feeling the deep pain I felt. That sounds very noble, but can you say God complex?

My heart and motives were pure. I just wanted to help those who were hurting, those whose choices and actions were leading them on a path of destruction. The problem is, I didn't have the ability to affect change. It's what I call passion without power. Therein lies the problem of stepping out where I've not been called to go.

For many years, I had a friend I felt passionately about helping. She was a single mom. She'd chosen to live as a single parent. She chose, with a vengeance, to be unhappy and bitter about it. I was bound and determined to help her overcome her bitterness and raise her child "right."

I invested years developing a friendship and providing a support system. At some point, I'm not really sure when, it became crystal clear I was trying to control her life. My heart had become overwhelmed with the pain of helping her change a life she obviously had no interest in changing. I had to let the friendship go for my own emotional well-being.

I've since realized that, although I couldn't change her, I might have been able to salvage the friendship if I could've changed my reaction to her. If I could've accepted her as she was.

Another friend lived an equally miserable existence but chose to stay in her marriage. She self-medicated with long work hours as an escape mechanism from the home she didn't want to be in. Again, I invested myself in "helping" her get her life in order and raise her children "right."

The moment of clarity came after years of seeing things weren't changing. Things weren't getting better. Once again, my heart became overwhelmed with the pain of helping her change a life she obviously had no interest in changing. Yet again, I realized I couldn't change her; I could only change my reaction to her. I needed to accept her right to make choices for her life.

In walks friend number three. I'm obviously a glutton for punishment or a very slow learner; I'm not sure which. Maybe both! My heart and motives were still pure; I just wanted to help. This friend had it all—looks, talent, charisma. She was well-liked, outgoing, and ever the optimist. That's where the illusion of perfection ends.

Like me, this friend had a burning desire to help people and became increasingly consumed with helping someone. I suppose that sounds a little funny coming from me. Judgmental for sure. My grandfather always told me, it takes one to know one. Oh, how right he was because that's when I saw it. My eyes were opened, and the truth became abundantly clear. I knew this consuming burden all too well.

The realization hit me square between the eyes as if I'd just been hit by an eighteen-wheeler. That truck didn't just hit me; it rolled over me, backed up, and roared right on over me again.

That comes close to describing the pain I felt when I realized I was once again trying to help people change lives they had no interest in changing. As miserable as I may have thought their lives were, they were their lives. I was trying to exert control where I had none. Passion without power.

Although each of these friendships has been lost or severely strained because of this powerless passion to fix other people's problems, my therapist has recently helped me put a name to what I was experiencing. It's called *codependency*.

That's right, I'm addicted to fixing other people's problems. That's the only explanation for how my life could be so affected by someone else's choices. I cared! I invested my heart, soul, and emotions into these friendships, into helping these people fix their lives. The day I had to make the choice to walk away from each of these relationships, which were toxic to me through no fault of theirs, a little piece of me died.

The natural reaction when we get hurt that badly is to think, I'll never do that again. I'll never care again. I'll never try to help someone again. It's too painful. However, not caring for people again, not trying to help them, is not an option for me. So what did I learn? How can I express this powerless passion without getting hurt in the process? I had to consider several things.

What do these three friends have in common? They've all chosen the life they're living. Whether happy or miserable through my lens, they've chosen it. How do the choices of these friends impact me? Well, if you ask my therapist, they don't; and actually, she's right. The reality remains I can't control people, places, things, or events. No matter how hard I try, this isn't something I'll ever be able to do.

Their choices about how to live their lives, whether good or bad from my perspective, can't hurt me. I'm not responsible for their happiness. Those last two sentences are profound. Why? They're profound because I didn't realize the simple truth of them until just a short time ago. They're so profound, I want to repeat them—other people's choices can't hurt me, because I'm not responsible for their happiness! I'm only responsible for my choices.

So, where did I go wrong? I chose to invest time, energy, and emotion into something I had absolutely no control over. Once again, passion without power. I'm not in control of their choices or their lives.

I can't control people, places, things, or events. No matter how hard I try, this isn't something I'll ever be able to do.

I can listen to them. I can be sad for them. I can love them. And I can pray for them. I can't change them. I must learn to accept them for who they are.

Just recently, when I was having my annual physical, I was sitting in the lab waiting to have my blood drawn. As I sat anxiously waiting for the lab tech to complete paperwork and pull all the beautifully colored vials that would eventually hold the precious blood about to be extracted from my unwilling veins, I saw a poster with the Serenity Prayer on the wall across from me.

I think most people know the Serenity Prayer. It's the foundation of any twelve-step program including, I discovered later, Co-Dependents Anonymous. I can quote it from memory.

However, it took on new meaning that day. Although I didn't actually see a lightbulb turn on above my head, the reaction I had to that quote was as clear to me as going from the darkness into the light.

I clearly wasn't accepting the things I couldn't change. I wasn't accepting my friends for who they'd chosen to be, who God had made them to be. I wanted them to be who I wanted them to be. Right then, I realized I needed help. As I researched the Serenity Prayer, I discovered the words people are familiar with are only a portion of the actual original prayer. The Serenity Prayer in its entirety is even more powerful.

I can only change myself. Let me allow that thought to hang there for a minute. Instead of trying to change everyone else, I need to invest that time, energy, and emotion into something I actually can change—me!

> **The Serenity Prayer**
>
> God grant me the serenity
> To accept the things I cannot change;
> Courage to change the things I can;
> And wisdom to know the difference.
> Living one day at a time;
> Enjoying one moment at a time;
> Accepting hardships as the pathway to peace;
> Taking, as He did, this sinful world as it is,
> Not as I would have it;
> Trusting that He will make all things right
> If I surrender to His Will;
> That I may be reasonably happy in this life
> And supremely happy with him forever in the next.
> Amen.
> (Niebuhr, 1932)

Regret – The Incurable Disease

Regret: those moments with my children I'll never be able to get back. Whether it be a rainy day I failed to grab a poncho and keep going or a thrilling coaster I didn't ride, I missed so many opportunities to create lasting memories with my children.

I cherish the memories I do have, all captured in photographs sorted neatly by year, and I wonder which memories should be there and aren't. I also remember vividly the day my youngest child turned eighteen and graduated from high school. I actually said to myself, "I can die happy now. I've done my job."

Regret: the friendships I've lost, or had to leave behind, because of a deep, burning desire to keep people from what I perceived as pain and suffering. The hours I invested attempting to help, with overwhelming love in my heart, I can now see as meddling with things that were none of my concern.

Regret: the small, seemingly insignificant moments where I chose a path that seemed right in my heart without looking to see if Jesus was out there on the water calling to me. How many opportunities did I miss because I didn't see him out there in the midst of a storm beckoning me to join him?

How many relationships did I mess up because I climbed out of that boat, certain I was needed, even if I couldn't see him calling me or didn't even take the time to look.

Doing Things God's Way

God doesn't want us to live a life of regret. God wants us to live a full and content life. Despite our circumstances, he is all we'll ever need, which is why he sent his son to pay the price for our sins. He wants us to cherish the moments we have with our family and friends just like he cherishes his moments with us.

He wants us to have the courage to get out of the boat and walk with him. The key here is walk *with* him. Peter was right when he heard those whispers of doubt saying people don't walk on water. They don't! People don't walk on water unless Jesus is with them.

Just like Peter, I need to learn to trust that if Jesus wants me to walk on water, he'll not only call me to step out of that boat, but he'll also control the waves.

I no longer want to live a life chained to fears, lies, and doubt.

I no longer want to, or feel the need to, be in control.

I no longer want to worry about things beyond my control, like falling from a roller coaster, rain on a special day, or saving the world.

Erroneously thinking I was in control all those years has only led to a life filled with stress, anxiety, sleepless nights, raw emotions, lost relationships, and bad choices.

Although my plans seemed well thought out and perfect based on my knowledge of the situation, God's plan is always better and considers things I

If he calls me, he'll calm the waves.

could never possibly think about. Isaiah 14:24 says, "As God plans, so shall it be."

It's even more clearly stated in Philippians 2:10: "At the name of Jesus *EVERY* knee *WILL* bow, of those who are in heaven and on earth and under the earth." (NASB, *emphasis mine*) We will end up acknowledging God is in control by choice now or by force in the end.

I choose to acknowledge God's control over every detail of my life, and everyone else's, starting right now. I know I'll have to recommit to this choice every time my flesh tries to slip back into control mode, and that won't be easy. But I make that commitment now. It's time. It's well past time, actually, for me to trust that God will call me out of the boat at the proper time. If he calls me, he'll calm the waves.

Inspiration Suggestions

➤ *We can make our plans, but God determines our steps. Proverbs 16:9*

➤ *Today I refuse to stress myself out about things I cannot control or change. Unknown*

➤ *Do not let what is out of your control interfere with all the things you can control. Unknown*

➤ *But when I am afraid, I will put my trust in you. Psalm 56:3*

➤ *Suffering arises from trying to control what is uncontrollable, or from neglecting what is within our power. Epictetus*

➤ *Remember who you are. Don't compromise for anyone, for any reason. You are a child of the Almighty God. Live that truth. Lysa Terkeurst*

➤ *Song – "Voice of Truth" by Casting Crowns**

➤ *Song – "I'm Letting Go" by Francesca Battistelli**

*Video available at https://bit.ly/2I38TXv

Reflect

1. Has control ever been taken from you unwillingly, leaving you hurt? What help are you getting to deal with that?

2. Do you ever lose control of your emotions—anger, fear, doubt?

3. What plans can you make for when that happens to stop the emotion cold in its track and put your focus back on God's power over your circumstances?

4. What opportunities have you missed out on because you were too afraid to step out of the boat?

5. What steps can you take now to build your faith and courage to avoid missing those opportunities in the future?

6. In what areas have you stepped out without being called and wreaked havoc in your life or in a relationship?

7. What steps can you take to give up control and restore those relationships?

8. After reading the description of codependency, do you think you may be codependent? In what ways? What can you do to give control back to whomever it belongs?

9. Were you familiar with the full Serenity Prayer? If not, how do you see it differently now in light of the additional verses?

10. In what ways do you need to start applying the Serenity Prayer to your life?

11. What regrets do you have about missed opportunities or missteps you've taken? What can you do to release those regrets?

12. What changes will you need to make so you are listening to God's call, responding appropriately, and making sure God is walking with you when you move?

13. What areas of your heart does God need to heal?

14. What destructive habits do you need to change?

15. Which Inspiration Suggestions did you choose to explore, and which stood out you'd like to remember?

16. What action steps do you need to take to implement what you've discovered in this chapter?

PART
II

How Do I Get Help?

5

I Need to Admit I Need Help

Surrendering

Okay. I get it. I've been trying to do it all for everyone except me. I've been trying to change it all in everyone except me. I've been trying to impress everyone, keep everyone happy, handle everything perfectly, control everything under the sun and for what possible reason?

When they feel bad, can't handle things, or just want to escape, some people turn to alcohol or drugs to self-medicate. In an attempt to escape my life, forget my past, and distract myself from my emotions, I chose to self-medicate as well.

I didn't do it with alcohol or drugs but with other people's problems and attempts to help them fix things. I filled my schedule with activities and responsibilities related to other people and my perception of their problems.

But the more I did, the worse I felt. I didn't need more. I just needed God. I needed him to fill me with his love so I could stop seeking approval from others. I needed him to increase my trust in him so I could stop trying to control everything. I needed him to heal all those wounds, strengthen my emotions, and give me the power to move forward. I needed to quit pretending things were fine and actually allow God to make them fine.

Quit Pretending

Years ago, my pastor asked me to share a brief testimony about my struggle with depression. I agreed, but I was terrified of the outcome. What if people didn't accept me anymore? What if, once they saw the real me, they walked away? What if...? That game could go on forever. In hindsight, it's easy to see these concerns as lies from the enemy.

How do I know that's what they were? I gave my testimony, or at least the reality of my depression at that point, and the response afterwards wasn't at all what I expected. It was like one of those social media videos that says, "You'll never believe what happened next!"

One of my friends who always looked so happy, pulled me aside and said, "Thank you! I never would've guessed you suffered from depression. You always look so happy." That's when I knew. He suffered from depression too. He told me as much as I listened to his story.

We were both doing the same thing. We were trying to fake happy until we felt happy. We may have been fooling the people around us, but we weren't fooling ourselves, and we certainly weren't fooling God. God knows everything.

Jeremy Camp's song "He Knows" reminds me God understands our suffering. He watched his only son suffer and die on the cross. Just like the weight of my depression overwhelms me and brings me to my knees, the weight of my sins brought Jesus to his knees.

With depression, if you fake it, you'll never make it. From my experience with depression, the only thing that works is face it and you'll make it.

Jesus knows how it feels because he felt it. He felt overwhelming pain, both physical and emotional, at a level I can't even fathom. The depth of despair I've felt at the worst moments of my depression are truly miniscule compared to the suffering Jesus experienced on the cross.

Does that mean my suffering doesn't matter? Absolutely not! Every detail of my life matters to God. He doesn't want me to suffer. He doesn't want anyone to suffer.

When Jesus met the woman at the well in John 4:1-26, he understood her suffering. He knew every detail of her life. He knew it and understood it, and he still met her there. Then he told her he was the antidote for the poison eating her from the inside out. He knew she wasn't fine. She was hiding and trying to escape her pain. She couldn't even face the other women from her village, so she came to the well alone.

Jesus asked her to give up all her struggles, to quit hiding, and to accept his help. Jesus couldn't make her past go away, but he could give her the freedom to live a new life, a different life in the future, free from the shame and despair she felt.

Just like that woman, I could only hide for so long before the truth started tumbling out. We've all heard the old adage "Fake it until you make it," but that doesn't always hold true. With depression, if you fake it, you'll never make it. From my experience with depression, the only thing that works is face it and you'll make it.

Jesus told that woman at the well he could give her a solution that would free her from her desperate life of shame and hiding forever. God is willing to do the same for each of us. He's willing to take away our shame and need for hiding if we will just surrender to him.

Coming to the Point of Surrender

My moment of surrender came a few years prior to sharing my testimony. I was taking a break from education and working in a home party plan business. I did well. I achieved top sales in my unit two years in a row and earned the use of a free car.

Yes, that really happens. Going to the dealership to pick up that shiny new red car was a feeling like no other. I was on top of the world. I finally felt like somebody.

But how easily it all came tumbling down. The use of that free car is only for two years. After that, if you don't requalify, the dealership comes to take it back. During my two years of free driving, God called me into service as a church secretary. Without a full-time focus on the business, I didn't requalify.

I'll never forget my overpowering despair as I stood in the front lobby of my church and watched out the glass doors as they drove off with my car. As I helplessly stood and watched, my pastor walked up behind me and asked if I was okay. I vividly remember even now the response I gave without even a single thought. I said, "Ever since I was raped, I've felt like a failure. Now I really am a failure."

The words slipped out before I realized what I was saying. Our families had been the closest of friends, and I'm sure he was shocked to hear this revelation he'd heard nothing about previously. I remember just staring at him for what seemed like a lifetime, trying to figure out what I'd just said that had him so confused.

That was the moment, two decades after it happened, I finally told someone other than my husband. He'd found out the hard way in a moment of passion when I had an intense flashback and almost clawed his eyes out. But this was the first admission to anyone else. That admission started a series of breakdowns and Band-Aid fixes littered over the next two decades.

When is enough really enough?

When do you say, "I'm done with this" and actually mean it?

When will you ever find the time to fix it, once and for all?

I didn't reach that point until two decades later when I truly couldn't imagine taking another breath in my current condition. All those years, God wanted to take it all away. God wanted to change my life. He wanted to soothe my soul.

All I had to do was ask. October 29, 2014, the day I experienced an emotional breakdown, is the day I finally did.

Fear of the Unknown

Once you ask God to help you, it's time to quit living in fear. 1 Samuel 17:32-51 tells us of a young boy who faced a similar situation and decided it was time to face his greatest fear.

David was the youngest of eight sons. He'd been anointed by the prophet, Samuel, to be the next king of Israel. From the day of his anointing, he grew deeply in spiritual knowledge and trust in God. While his older brothers were at war, David was relegated to going back and forth between tending his father's sheep and serving in the temple with the current king, Saul.

On the battlefield, his older brothers faced what appeared to be an overwhelming challenge every day for forty days. That challenge was a giant named Goliath. All the soldiers ran in fear from Goliath's taunts.

The king became dismayed when none of his mighty warriors would take on this bully, so he offered up a reward for the man courageous enough to defeat Goliath.

Still, none of the warriors would face off against Goliath. Those warriors chose to live in misery and humiliation rather than step out and trust God to change things. I completely understand since I was doing the same thing. For two decades after I admitted my rape and started seeking help, I also lived in misery and humiliation, too afraid to trust God to fix it.

David was different. He came to the battlefield one day bringing supplies. There, he overheard the dilemma the king's warriors were facing. He was outraged that Goliath was attempting to humiliate his God and God's people.

His brothers, along with the entire army, laughed when David, a lowly shepherd, suggested he would defeat Goliath. He said, "The Lord who rescued me from the paw of the lion and the paw of the bear; he will rescue me from the hand of this Philistine." (1 Samuel 17:37) David chose to trust God even when the warriors didn't.

The warriors knew the life of a shepherd was no training for a boy about to face an oversized soldier with a lifetime of military experience. And they were right.

On his own, David could never have defeated Goliath. When he put the military equipment on, he almost fell over from the weight and bulkiness of it. It was too much for him to carry alone. He wasn't used to the tools of war.

But he trusted God, and that's what spurred him into action. He knew this enemy of the Israelites was an enemy of God. He was determined to stop him.

David's only battle experience was defeating wild animals who preyed on the flock he tended. He did so simply with the tools God provided at the time of the threat. So now, as he faced Goliath, David looked around for a tool to use. All he saw were several smooth stones. He wasn't sure how they would defeat a giant, but he picked some up.

With unwavering confidence based on a solid trust in God to overcome this new enemy as he had all the others, David approached Goliath. He defeated him with just those few smooth stones. Once again, God had provided a way to defeat his enemy.

He had no fear about facing an unknown enemy. He simply knew, based on his experiences with God in the past, that God would defeat whatever obstacle stood in his way. There was never a question of whether he could defeat Goliath, only the knowledge he would.

When we face our giant—depression—fear builds within us. We just can't defeat it. We've tried before. Our past tells us there's no point in trying; we can't succeed.

However, what if our past had been like David's? What if we knew with certainty God would defeat our enemy? If I'd known God could overcome my pain, hurt, and terribly messed up life, I would have let him decades earlier than I did.

Okay, that's probably not a fair statement. I knew he could; I just wasn't willing to admit I couldn't. I wasn't ready to give up trying to fix it on my own.

Paul indicates that although we are pressed on all sides, we will not be crushed. Even though we are hunted down, we will never be abandoned or alone. Even when we feel struck down, we can be assured we will not be destroyed. (2 Corinthians 4:8-9)

That all sounds great, and it's true. However, I did feel crushed. I also felt alone and destroyed. It wasn't until the weight of my depression forced me so far down I was sure I couldn't possibly survive that I was willing to admit defeat.

God was my help. God wanted to provide small, smooth stones for me to throw at my giant, if I would just let him.

Time to Surrender

After my breakdown, when I found myself sitting alone in the hospital staring at the zip ties that replaced my shoelaces, I realized I'd finally hit rock bottom. It was abundantly clear these people believed I could no longer be trusted to take care of my own life.

I didn't know what else to do but pray. As I sat there trying to find the words to say, I remembered the words of the song "Just Say Jesus." I just needed to cry out the name of Jesus. Nothing more.

He knew everything already. He knew what I needed. Asaph, a musician at the time David was king over Israel, probably expressed it better than I could. He said, "My health fails; my spirits droop, yet God remains! He is the strength of my heart; he is mine forever!" (Psalm 73:26, LB)

Seeking God at that moment was the first step in the right direction for me. Even though that dreary hospital room and those revealing zip ties certainly didn't look or feel like the right direction, I knew God was with me.

For the first time in my adult life, God was leading the way. I truly wasn't in charge of my life. My therapist has since reminded me that fear can have two meanings: Forget Everything And Run or Face Everything And Recover. All I knew at that lonely moment in my room was that I was tired of running. For the first time, I truly wanted nothing more than to recover.

There are interventions for addicts who want to recover. Why are there no interventions for those who are depressed? Why are we, as a society, so afraid of confronting mental illness? Until you reach the breaking point, as I did, you often suffer in silence.

I suffered silently with depression for forty years, so I sat in that hospital room filled with regret. The intense pain I suffered over the next few months as I started my recovery was certainly difficult, but it was also temporary. The regret I feel over what might have been is forever.

Only God can heal that wound, and he wants to heal it. Jesus was wounded and died centuries ago so I might not have to suffer. He declared victory on my behalf long before I was even born. Just like David, all I had to do was believe my giant would certainly be defeated. I had to start living victoriously.

To gloss over the suffering part of my current victory would be a disservice. We'll talk later about how to survive this intensely painful and overwhelmingly difficult recovery phase. But for now, just know God is waiting to walk with you—hand in hand.

Believe me when I say I would never have stopped staring at those zip ties and gotten off that bed if God hadn't gently taken my hand and said, "Come to me all you who are weary and burdened and I will give you rest." (Matthew 11:28)

Of course, I had to make the choice to go with him; and I have to make the decision daily to stand firm in that choice. I can rest knowing God will defeat all my enemies if I will place my trust in him.

God is waiting patiently for us to give up and ask for his help. He doesn't just want us to look fine; he wants us to actually be fine. It's time. Cry out to Jesus and take that first step with him.

Inspiration Suggestions

➢ *I have been driven many times upon my knees by the overwhelming conviction that I had nowhere else to go. My own wisdom and that of all about me seemed insufficient for that day. Abraham Lincoln*

➢ *God always has and always will look for men and women who say to him, "I trust you so much, I'm all in. I want your way not mine. I am willing to live by faith!" Chip Ingram*

➢ *I am simply not enough in myself, but in Him I am. This surrender is not weakness, but the only true measure of strength any of us have. Aaron W. Matthews*

➢ *Father, if you are willing, please take this cup of suffering away from me. Yet I want your will to be done, not mine. Luke 22:32*

➢ *When we choose to surrender our mind to God, he will honor that choice and give us the strength and power to think right. Mary Southerland*

➢ *Sometimes surrender means giving up from trying to understand and becoming comfortable with not knowing. Eckhart Tolle*

➢ *Trust in the Lord with all your heart; do not depend on your own understanding. Seek his will in all you do, and he will show you which path to take. Proverbs 3:5-6*

➢ *Song – "Tell Your Heart to Beat Again" by Danny Gokey**

➢ *Song – "Oh My Soul" by Casting Crowns**

➢ *Song – "Just Be Held" by Casting Crowns**

➢ *Song – "Even If" by Mercy Me**

➢ *Song – "Thy Will" by Hillary Scott & the Scott Family**

*Video available at https://bit.ly/2I38TXv

Reflect

1. Do you self-medicate to avoid what's causing you pain? If so, with what?

2. In what ways is self-medicating only making matters worse?

3. Are you trying to fake happy until you feel happy?

4. Have you been hiding and avoiding others like the woman at the well?

5. Do you believe God doesn't understand your pain? Do you believe even he can't help you?

6. Have you experienced that moment when you said, "Enough! I'm not doing this anymore"? Have you been there more than once?

7. What will it take to say those words and actually mean it? To actually start the journey to recovery?

8. What would it take for you to surrender your pain and trust God can heal you?

9. Does your history tell you you'll never be able to defeat your depression?

10. Do you have enough faith to believe God can overcome any giant?

11. Do you believe God loves you enough to overcome your giant, depression? Are you ready to trust him to do it?

12. Which Inspiration Suggestions did you choose to explore, and which stood out you'd like to remember?

13. What action steps do you need to take to implement what you've discovered in this chapter?

6

I Need to Understand I'm Never Alone

Seeking Out Spiritual Support

Is "one" really the loneliest number? Only if I look around me instead of inside of me. There may not be any people physically around me, or anyone I feel close to emotionally, but I'm never truly alone. God is always with me. Just because I can't feel him nearby, or I feel like he's deserted me, doesn't mean he isn't working in the background.

I can't see or feel electricity working in the background either (unless, of course, I touch something I shouldn't), but the power company is always working behind the scenes to keep everything up and running. Similarly, I can't see the wind (unless it turns into a hurricane), but I know it's always there.

In an actual hurricane, when the wind knocks out my electricity, I have no power to accomplish the things I normally do in my everyday life. Suddenly, even simple things become difficult and draining. However, I know the power company is already aware of my problem and working on it. Their electricians and lineman are probably on it before I even get a chance to call for help. They work as quickly as safety allows to get my power working again. They don't want me to suffer without power. God feels the same way about me and my life.

Sometimes, I have hurricanes in my personal life unrelated to wind or weather. When a big life storm hits, like serious medical issues or financial problems, I get knocked down. I struggle with even the simplest tasks of everyday life. I find myself wondering where I can find help.

Then I remember, "My help comes from the Lord, the Maker of heaven and earth." (Psalm 121:2) That's right; the God who created the universe cares enough about me to help with any problem I might have on any given day.

Just like the power company, God is watching over me and is aware of my problem even before I am. God wants me to make that call for help to say the storms in my life have knocked me out, to recognize I can't fix things on my own. I need the help God provides! I need my power turned back on. Fortunately, I know how to reach him.

Returning to God (or Realizing My Need for Him)

As I sat in that hospital room hour after hour too afraid to even go out into the hall where there were people, it sank into my dense brain matter that I had nowhere to go. I felt like I had nowhere to turn. I felt alone in the universe. I was the proverbial "one" that felt so lonely.

To my left was a completely sealed opaque window. Ahead of me was a bathroom with no lock on the door and a shelf holding my belongings. To my right was another bed, empty for the moment, and a door. That door led to the big, bad, scary world I was afraid to face.

I sat there alone with my thoughts. I had nothing, and I had nowhere I wanted to go badly enough to put my feet on the floor beside my bed. So, I sat there. Alone. I had no one to help me.

Or did I?

I stared at that shelf ahead of me, holding the only belongings I had been allowed to keep: a few shirts, sweatpants with the strings removed, undergarments with underwires removed, a toothbrush, toothpaste, a comb, shampoo, and my Bible.

Why, when the doctor told my husband to take me to the hospital, had I thought to grab my Bible? It was apparent I had a connection to this book far beyond what I currently felt as I looked back at that hallway door. Beyond it were people, people locked in a mental health hospital. The doors at either end of the short hallway were locked. They were locked to keep these people in. They were locked to keep me in. I slowly realized I was now one of them.

I didn't want to be one of those people. I wanted to be well. I wanted to stop hurting. I wanted to stop running. Gradually, I concluded that if I truly wanted to stop running, the window on the left and the hallway on the right were no longer an option. I knew if I really did want to get well, to stop hurting, to stop running, I had to stay right where I was. I had to face my issues. I had to find someone to help me. But where?

I stared at my Bible. Again, I pondered why I had brought it. Somehow, something deep inside me knew that Bible was where the answers lay. Inside my Bible was the someone I needed to help me. There were plenty of doctors, psychiatrists, and therapists in that hospital. I needed more. I needed what only that Bible could offer—the source of my personal power!

When Life's Little Hurricanes Strike

I was in the midst of my own personal hurricane. In fact, I was in the eye of the storm. Hurricanes are very common where I live in Florida, so I've learned a lot about them. The eye of a hurricane is the very center of the storm where everything is calm and quiet. On a weather map, the eye of the hurricane is the beautiful, blue sky circle in the midst of the larger circle of white storm clouds. The winds and destruction circulate around this center point. I have heard it's so eerily quiet you can hear your own heart beating.

There is one common characteristic in the center of anything—it marks the halfway point. Although in the center of the hurricane it seems quiet and peaceful, history tells us the destruction is going to start up again any second, ravaging everything around it again, until the storm slowly moves completely away.

In that silent moment in the eye of this life storm, I made a decision. There was no escape from the hospital bed I found myself on, and I knew the second half of this storm was still coming.

However, I also knew that just as a physical hurricane has a landfall, an eye, and an end, my storm would end as well. My storm would eventually move completely away, leaving calm blue skies in its wake. I knew for the time being though, I had to shelter in place. That's a time when it's too late to avoid the storm. The only safe option is to ride it out where you are. That hospital bed represented the only safe place for me in this particular storm.

As I started to think clearly for the first time in decades, I somehow knew the only way to ride out this storm, the only way to eliminate the pain, was to stop trusting in my own efforts and trust in God. I knew I couldn't stop the pain any more than I could stop an actual hurricane. I also knew for certain God could stop the pain if he chose to do so.

However, even if God chose not to stop my pain, I knew with certainty he could give me the strength to withstand it. I knew my God was able! (Romans 16:25)

I looked at that Bible and remembered all the stories where God was able to overcome what we consider overwhelming odds, and I knew he could be trusted to do it again. I knew God wouldn't let the pain overcome me. I knew he would keep me safe. I knew the words in that Bible of mine declared over and over again the promises of God to protect me and make me victorious. From Genesis to Revelation, God's character never changes. If I continued to fight, with God as my strength, I would eventually overcome my depression.

It wasn't easy at that moment to concede there was no hope for me without God's strength. Remember, I'm a problem solver. I fix things. But I couldn't fix this. I had messed up my life and, without God, I had no power to fix it. Why had I not trusted God all along?

The moment I conceded my powerlessness, and acknowledged God's power, was better than the Hallelujah chorus to God. For when one sinner repents and cries out for help, all of heaven rejoices. (Luke 15:7)

Right then, I repented. I cried out once again to my God for help. This time, I heard him. I didn't hear an audible voice, but I heard God speak very clearly. He said, "I am here! I am with you!"

I knew he was with me. I could feel his presence as surely as I felt each of my babies, whom I couldn't see or hear, kick my belly. My fear subsided. My view of what was to come in my future brightened. I knew without question God held my life in his hands. Because God sent Jesus to save me, no matter how terrifying my future seemed at that moment, I knew it was worth it to continue fighting.

I suddenly had somewhere to go badly enough to put my feet on the ground beside that bed. I walked over to the shelf holding my every possession and picked up my Bible. I sat back down on that hospital bed and started to read, knowing for certain I would find what I needed.

My friend Emily once asked for help finding something she needed. She had recently moved, with the help of many others, as she was with her son in the hospital. The problem was, she couldn't find some critical paperwork she needed. She'd torn into every box and couldn't locate the paperwork in any of them. My motto is always, "Nothing is ever lost until Momma can't find it." Knowing that, she sought my assistance in finding the paperwork. We knew those papers had to be there. And they were important enough that she couldn't go on without finding them. They had to be found! So, we set out to find those papers as if our lives depended on it. In this case, hers pretty much did.

We eventually found the paperwork. We found it because we unleashed a determination and focus like never before. We put aside everything else until those papers were found.

As I sat in that hospital room, I realized it was time to release that same determination and focus on finding a way to overcome my depression. I knew I couldn't do it on my own. I knew only God's power could. I also knew the Bible held the answers.

God was with me. I was sure of it. Although I felt the peace of God's presence and knew I needed to trust him, I was having trouble trusting a God I felt like I barely knew.

Getting to Know God

I certainly thought I knew God. I had believed *in* him all my life. I believed he existed. I believed all my sins from the past were forgiven. I believed he helped people. I just didn't believe he could, or would, help me. That was the first time I realized I didn't really *know* him. It wasn't how much I knew *about* God that mattered. It was how much I actually *knew* God. I couldn't trust someone I didn't know. I had to figure out who God really was before I could not only believe *in* him, I could *believe* him. I needed to finally believe his promises were true for me! So, how did I get to really know God?

Reading/Hearing God's Word. God's Word is alive and active. It's so powerful it can divide soul from spirit, joint from marrow, and judge the motives in our heart. No one can hide from him. Our lives are naked and open before him to whom we must give account. (Hebrews 4:12-13) These verses point out the precision with which God can see into our lives, and the intensity with which we need to allow his Word to sink into our lives.

Like a surgeon can swiftly and precisely open up our heart, diagnose disease, and lay out a treatment plan for restoring health, God's Word can expose a lack of spiritual health within us. He can then reveal his treatment plan for restoring us to him. Getting to know who God is—his character, his traits, his plan—required me to spend time in his Word.

I knew my Bible, which had been sitting on that sparsely occupied shelf, held an entire history of man and the involvement of God in their lives. It also held the treatment plan perfect for my spiritual health condition, which I knew for certain was the cause of my current physical/mental health condition.

In addition to the Bible, music has always been a way in which God has revealed himself and his character to me. In "He Is," Aaron Jeoffrey breaks the Bible down to the book level, sharing the sixty-six names by which God's people knew him. Whenever I hear this song performed live, the entire room rises to their feet in applause as its powerful message draws to an end. Another moving song that outlines the names and characteristics of God is "I Am" by Mark Schultz.

The Bible and Christian music are only two methods of getting into God's Word. Weekly Sunday morning messages, church small groups, Christian Life books, devotionals, and Christian conferences all provide a look into God's Word. Another way to get to know God is through prayer.

> *Getting to know who God is—his character, his traits, his plan—required me to spend time in his Word.*

Praying God's Word. God knows exactly what you need even before you ask. (Matthew 6:7-8) In the verses following this, Jesus goes on to teach us how to pray. The Lord's Prayer teaches us to pray from a point of personal relationship with God, with respect and reverence for his power, submission to his will, as well as trust in and dependence on his provision.

Have you ever had a friend you could trust and depend on no matter what? This type of friend is rare. It generally takes years to reach a level of intimacy this deep. God wants to be that kind of friend to you. He wants to have such a close personal relationship that talking to him and sharing everything with him happens without thought. It is times like the one I was experiencing, where I felt completely lost and alone, when this type of friendship with God is so critical.

Again, music played a role in reminding me that, although I was physically by myself in that room, I wasn't alone. I can always share my deepest fears and emotions with God. I'm reminded just exactly what a privilege that is in "What a Friend We Have in Jesus." We can pour out our broken heart; we can ask for our heart's true desire. We can even just cry out the name of Jesus. God already knows it all. He knows what we need. He just wants us to talk to him, to love him, and to trust him.

Many people say they can't pray because they don't know what to say. They feel a little weird speaking honestly about their needs and desires with God. Many well-known Christian speakers have written on the topic of praying God's Word.

What a Friend We Have in Jesus

What a friend we have in Jesus, all our sins and grief to bear.
What a privilege to carry everything to God in prayer.
Oh what peace we often forfeit, oh what needless pain we bear.
All because we do not carry everything to God in prayer.

Have we trials and temptations?
Is there trouble anywhere?
We should never be discouraged – take it to the Lord in prayer.
Can we find a friend so faithful, who will all our sorrows share?
Jesus knows our every weakness; take it to the Lord in prayer.

Are we weak and heavy-laden, cumbered with a load of care?
Precious Savior, still our refuge – take it to the Lord in prayer.
Do thy friends despise, forsake thee? Take it to the Lord in prayer.
In His arms He'll take and shield thee, Thou wilt find a solace there.

Blessed Savior, Thou hast promised Thou will all our burdens bear.
May we ever, Lord, be bringing all to thee in earnest prayer.
Soon in glory bright, unclouded, there will be no need for prayer.
Rapture, praise, and endless worship will be our sweet portion there.

Joseph M. Scriven, 1855

Praying God's Word means speaking words of truth from the Bible back to God. God makes many promises in the Bible we can apply to our lives.

Remember what we discussed earlier—repentance means agreeing with God your life isn't in line with his will. Praying God's Word is similar. It involves agreeing God's promises are in line with his will for our life, and, therefore, desiring to see those promises fulfilled in our life.

Some theologians believe we can't take every promise in the Bible and apply it to our lives randomly. Some promises are specific to a person or nation, not universal. I believe that's true.

I'm by no means a theologian, and I'm certainly not here to debate that point. What I do know to be true is that God's character never changes. Every book I read throughout the Bible shows God time and again making a promise and keeping it. In my mind, that assures me God will keep his promises to love me, protect me, and bring me safely home to him, if I will love him and surrender to his will.

That's the hard part—surrendering to his will.

I found myself realizing in that quiet moment that I wanted to surrender to his will. I wanted to pray his promises back to him, but I also realized I couldn't pray God's Word back to him if I didn't know God's Word. This sent me straight back to reading/hearing God's Word. It was time for me to get into that Bible and study his Word, his promises. That's when things started to change.

Growing in God's Word. "Show me the right path, O Lord; point out the road for me to follow. Lead me by your truth and teach me, for you are the God who saves me. All day long I put my hope in you." (Psalm 25:4-5) This verse points out the first step I needed to take, which was to allow God to point me towards the path he had planned for me long ago, the path I clearly wasn't following. At that moment, I could clearly see which path I was on, and which one I was supposed to be on. I got it. Find path. Check!

Next, I needed to allow God to teach me how to follow his path through the truth revealed in his Word. I needed to follow his directions for how to get from where I was to where I wanted to go. Correction—where HE wanted me to go. It wasn't enough to realize I was on the wrong path; I needed to also realize I was trying to navigate it on my own.

When I was a young driver, navigating on your own was the only way to get from point A to point B. You had to look at maps and get directions. There was no automatic GPS. Inevitably, it was the fourth right instead of the third right or exit 192B not 192A. Or we were so busy talking and admiring the scenery that we missed the exit entirely even though we knew where to turn.

I got lost, a lot, and made numerous U-turns to get to my final destination.

Now, while driving, I use a GPS navigation system. It always gets me where I want to go.

My eighty-year-old electronically challenged mother, on the other hand, continued to drive using maps and directions. I escorted her into the twenty-first century by convincing her to try a GPS navigation system when driving.

At first, she rebelled, announcing, "This is not the right way to go." She wanted to continue using her sense of direction rather than trust that the GPS knew what it was talking about. Then she would angrily fuss at the system for telling her to "make a U-turn," or "return to the route."

A few months after my father passed away, my mother decided to navigate her way from Missouri to Florida to visit me for Christmas. I helped her program her daily start and stop points in the system, avoiding Atlanta at all cost, and trusted she would be fine.

Day one – no problems. She made it through busy Memphis without any problems and arrived safely at her hotel for the night. She was happy and relaxed when she called to say she was settled in for the night. She even commented she was excited about her little adventure.

Day two – no problems. She found her way down into southern Mississippi and found a nice place to spend the night. Again, a relaxed, happy call to announce her day's success.

Day three – you knew it couldn't last forever, right? She called me midday and with a slightly nervous tone announced, "I'm fine. The car is fine. But I'm stuck in the middle of the highway, and everyone is just stopped. Some people are turning around in a wooded area off the road. Should I do that?"

What?

I told her to stay put and under no circumstances to turn around in the woods. I was able to go onto the Highway Patrol site and discovered that a tractor-trailer had gone over the side of an overpass, causing the cab to crash to the road below and sending a ball of flames covering the highway above. The trailer, which remained on the highway, had tipped over, spewing debris all over the highway. (Insert deep sigh of relief she was not involved and was safe)

While she waited, she tried to program a new route into the GPS system. No such luck. It completely shut down. It apparently was finished working so hard.

After a two-hour delay on the highway, she was able to safely navigate on her own to a stopping point for the night in the panhandle of Florida. The phone call at the end of this day had a different tone than the first two days: anxiety, exhaustion, and confusion.

Day four – The GPS system apparently decided it needed another day of vacation. My adventurous mother took off on her own, thinking she knew how to get the rest of the way through Florida, since she and my father wintered in Florida for many years. Smooth sailing then, right?

Enter stage left—Jacksonville. Again, I get a call midday, "I'm ok. The car is ok. I just don't know where I am." She had missed the cut-off to bypass Jacksonville and head south to my house. She was lost. She was navigating on her own and ended up in places she didn't expect. The good news is, she arrived safely later that day, but she swore she would never do it again.

The thing my mother liked best about her GPS system was how it gave her advance warning to make sure she didn't miss things. It doesn't say, "In 1,400 miles you will be at your destination." It says, "In 1.5 miles, turn left." It knows the entire route, but it takes her one step at a time. She doesn't know what's coming after that left turn 1.5 miles up the road. She learned to trust that her GPS knows and will tell her after she is obedient with the first direction. And luckily for my mother, and all of us, God never stops working like my mom's GPS did. We can trust he is always there to give the next direction if we are willing to listen.

Getting to Know God

As I think about this little adventure, I realize it's exactly what I was trying to do with my life. I started off on the right road with clear directions to my final destination. I was happy and on track. Then life happened. My internal GPS was still working, unlike my mother's on the last part of her trip, but I had quit listening. I had decided I could navigate on my own. I was following my own GPS instead of God's GPS.

Just as my mother's adventure became chaotic without her guidance system, my life had turned to chaos without mine. God knew where he wanted to take me, but without him directing my path, step by step, I got lost.

Growing with God requires me to recognize the right path, which I had figured out as I sat in that lonely hospital room. Remember? Find path. Check! But it also requires me to let God lead me on that path. I had to quit trying to navigate my life on my own. My guidance system sat right there in front of me. My little Bible held all the answers I needed. It held the truth about God, my navigator. It held the truth of who God is and what he expects from me on this journey of life.

> With the Lord's authority I say this: Live no longer as the Gentiles do, for they are hopelessly confused. Their minds are full of darkness; they wander far from the life God gives because they have closed their minds and hardened their hearts against him. They have no sense of shame. They live for lustful pleasure and eagerly practice every kind of impurity. But that isn't what you learned from Christ. Since you have heard about Jesus and have learned the truth that comes from him, throw off your old sinful nature and your former way of life, which is corrupted by lust and deception. Instead, let the Spirit renew your thoughts and attitudes. Put on your new nature, created to be like God – truly righteous and holy. (Ephesians 4:17-24)

These verses are very clear about what God expects of me now that I know the truth of his Word. He expects me to leave my old life behind, to change. He wants me to stop acting like a spoiled two-year-old who always wants, and usually gets, her own way. In other words, he expects me to grow up and leave the self-centered the-world-exists-to-please-me mindset behind. He expects me to become mature in my view of the world and my role in it.

Studying, learning, and knowing the truth is the easy part. It's time-consuming, no doubt, but easy, nonetheless. Actually growing and making changes in our lives based on that truth is where the work really starts. That requires trust. Trust in God to lead you step by step, turn by turn, without seeing what is ahead. Be obedient to the first direction he gives you, and then he will give you another.

God Is the Same Yesterday, Today, and Tomorrow

When my father passed away a few months ago, I walked out behind the casket with my mother and sister. My father was in heaven. Of that, there was no doubt. Yet, as we approached the vehicle that would take him away forever, I became completely overwhelmed with emotion. I felt like I couldn't breathe or even stand up at the thought of never being able to see him, or hug him, or hear his many jokes.

Suddenly, I realized I couldn't take another breath or even another step without God's help. I stood where I was and just began crying out to God. I couldn't even find the words, so I just started repeating all the things I knew to be true about God. All the characteristics of God that will never change. They were true that day in my hospital room, they were true at that moment as I watched the casket being taken away, they are true as I sit and write this, and they will be true forever.

God never changes.

He was the same yesterday as he is today. He will be the same forever.

Attributes of God Cheat Sheet

As an educator, I always liked to help my students by providing what I affectionately called a cheat sheet. It helped them remember things that were important, things they might need to know when a test came. Those characteristics of God couldn't have come rolling out of my mouth on that day if they hadn't been put there for safekeeping long before they were ever needed.

To get you started storing up these attributes of God now, and for future use when life throws a pop quiz your way, I've compiled a list of the attributes of God. I've summarized so they're easy to read and remember. However, I encourage you to read the scripture in its entirety for context and study purposes.

God Loves Me	
John 1:12	**I am a child of God**. (I am accepted even in my imperfection and I am loved. God loves me in an even greater way than I love my children. Even when my children mess up, I wait patiently to

	pick up the pieces. I may be disappointed in them, but I still love them.)
John 3:16	**God gave his one and only son for me.** (Imagine offering up your own child's life in exchange for someone who ignores you and complains all the time. He loves me that much!)
1 John 4:16	**I can rely on God's love for me.** (Once I acknowledge Jesus as my savior because of his sacrifice on the cross, I can trust in the love God has for me.)
God Knows Me	
Isaiah 43:1-2	**God knows my name.** (He paid the ransom to free me from captivity to my sins. I'm his.)
Matthew 6:7-8	**God knows exactly what I need before I ask.** (I don't need to use fancy language or lengthy prayers. I can simply call out the name of Jesus.)
John 4:16-18	**God knows me personally.** (God knows everything we've done past and present. Nothing is a surprise to him.)
Ephesians 1:11	**God chose me and has a plan for my life.** (We were chosen by God and appointed to fulfill his specific purpose for our lives. All before we were even born.)
1 John 3:20	**God is greater than my emotions.** (Our hearts and minds may accuse us and make us feel guilty, but the truth is God is bigger than any of that.)
God Hears Me	
Exodus 3:7-8	**God is aware of my suffering.** (God hears me when I cry out for help, and he desires to rescue me.)
Psalm 18:6	**God answers me when I cry out.** (The God of the universe who sits in heaven personally responds to my cries for help. He doesn't always give the answer I hope, but he always answers.)
1 John 5:14	**God hears when I ask in his name.** (I can ask

	with confident expectation when I know my request is in line with God's will for me.)
God Is My Deliverer/Savior/Redeemer	
Psalm 34:17-19	**God will deliver me from trouble**. (As a Christ-follower, I will face many difficulties in my life, but God will be there to rescue me every time.)
John 3:16	**God is my Savior and Redeemer**. (Jesus died on the cross to pay for the sins I have committed. I was bought with a price—the blood of Jesus.)
John 8:12	**Jesus is the light of the world**. (Without Jesus, I walk in the darkness of my own sin. Jesus provides the light for me to follow in a world still walking in darkness.)
John 6:48	**Jesus is the bread of life**. (Jesus' death gives me life. Without him I can't survive.)
John 11:25	**Jesus is the resurrection and the Life**. (If I believe in and rely on Jesus, I may die a physical death, but spiritually I will live forever.)
John 14:6	**Jesus is the way, the truth, and the life**. Enough said.
Romans 8:1-4	**God will not condemn me**. (Because I accept the payment for my sins Jesus provided, I live by the Holy Spirit's power within me. I've been set free from the sin and death the law requires.)
Revelation 1:18	**God holds the keys of death and Hades**. (While Jesus died on the cross, he also rose from the dead and is alive today in heaven. Death and Hades couldn't contain him. God alone holds the keys to free me as well.)
God Is My Helper/Strengthener	
Psalm 46:1-2	**God is there when I need him**. (I don't need to fear, no matter what the circumstances around me. God will give me the strength to overcome.)
Psalm 62:8	**God is my helper**. (I can confidently trust in him and rely on him despite what I'm going through.)

Isaiah 41:14	**God will help me.** (No matter how badly I mess up, I'm God's child. He saved me. He *will* help me!)
Habakkuk 3:19	**God is my strength.** (When I feel fear, want to give up, or am unable to even stand, God makes me brave and strong against any foe.)
Ephesians 3:20	**God is able.** (Through the power of the Holy Spirit living within me, God can make anything happen in my life, no matter how overwhelming it seems.)
God Is My Protector	
Genesis 15:1	**God calms my fears.** (When I question God's plan, or question the circumstances surrounding me, God reminds me there is no need to be afraid. He's got this.)
Deuteronomy 31:8	**God goes before me.** (When I face a battle in my life, God will walk in front of me, beside me, and behind me, sacrificing himself so that I might live. He's my own personal secret service agent.)
Romans 8:31-33	**God is on my side.** (If God gave up his only son to save me, he'll do everything necessary to keep me safe, so I can spend eternity with him.)
Romans 8:35	**God will always be with me.** (Though friends and family may turn away when I face tough times, God loves me, and he'll never turn away.)
2 Thessalonians 3:16	**God is peace.** (Because my salvation is secure, I already know how the story ends. I may have ups and downs in life, but peace can surround me, as I know how it will all turn out.)
God Is My Conqueror/Overcomer	
Luke 18:27	**God makes everything possible.** (Just because I can't do something, haven't ever seen it happen, or the world tells me it simply can't be done, doesn't mean it's impossible.)
1 John 5:3-5	**God helps me overcome the world.** (My faith in, and reliance on, the truth of Christ's sacrifice

	at the cross for me provides the power of the Holy Spirit in my life to conquer whatever obstacles I face.)
2 Corinthians 4:8-9	**God will not let anything defeat me**. (No matter what comes my way, it will not destroy me. I may be surrounded by trouble, in fear for my life, confused and dismayed, but God is there. Though I may lose the current battle, I *will* win the war.)
God Is My Provider	
Genesis 22:12-14	**God will provide**. (When I offer my life up for God's purposes and try to obey his every command, he'll provide everything I need.)
Psalm 23:1	**God provides, I lack nothing**. (God looks over me and gives me everything I need.)
John 15:5	**God is the vine, I am the branch**. (Just as a rose cut from a bush can live for only a short time, when I cut myself off from a relationship with God, I also can't survive.)
God Is Stable/He Never Changes	
Revelation 1:8	**God is the beginning and the end**. (God was here when the universe was created, and he'll be here when the universe is gone. God controls everything.)
Revelation 1:18	**God lives forever**. (Death couldn't contain him. He is alive today and will be long after I depart this earth.)
God Is Always With Me/God Is the Giver of Second Chances	
Psalm 66:20	**God will never reject my prayer or withhold his love**. (Friends, and even family, may lose interest in hearing about my struggles or caring for me in times of extended need. God will never ignore me. He will love and care for me forever.)
Psalm 86:15	**God is merciful and patient**. (Sometimes I become irritable and allow the troubles I'm facing to make me less than desirable to be

	around. God doesn't get angry with me for acting out or complaining. His patience in unending. He always forgives.)
John 16:7-8	**God has sent me a helper.** (When I accept Jesus' death on my behalf, God sends the Holy Spirit to help me overcome the temptations of my flesh, so I can keep his laws and be made righteous when his judgment comes.)
1 John 1:9	**God will forgive me if I repent.** (I must confess my sins by admitting to God I know my motives, thoughts, and/or actions were wrong. The world may find me guilty, but God will always find me not guilty.)
God Is Faithful & Trustworthy/Keeps His Promises	
Deuteronomy 7:6-9	**God keeps his promises.** (God chose me to be his child. Just as I have seen him do for his children throughout the Bible, I know I can trust him to keep his promises to me.)
Psalm 9:8-10	**God has never abandoned those who chase after him.** (God will judge right from wrong. If I earnestly seek him to save me from the judgment and give me the strength to live by his laws and not be led by fleshly desires, he won't leave me to die.)
Psalm 105:8	**God keeps his promises.** (The promise he made to his people is always at the forefront of God's mind. He will never break it.)
2 Corinthians 1:21-22	**God sent the Holy Spirit just as he promised.** (The Holy Spirit and the spiritual gifts we have received from God are but a portion of his promise to us. Because we know he is faithful, we can be certain he will stand up to what he promised.)

God Is Always with Me

In the storm, I called out and God heard me. He convinced me he had a perfect plan and he could be trusted. Now that I'm committed to following his guidance system instead of mine, I do believe his way was better all along. I know that no matter what I've faced in the past, or what I will face in the future, God is always with me. I know even though the unknown is a big, scary place, God will walk with me, and nothing can hurt me as long as I surrender to his will for my life.

> *I know that no matter what I've faced in the past, or what I will face in the future, God is always with me.*

Just like that hurricane, after it has moved on to terrorize somewhere else, the bright, sunny sky in its wake reveals the truth—sometimes things get destroyed. My old life needed to be destroyed. I needed it to be over. I needed to rebuild from the ground up. In the same way, after the hurricane is gone, lives are changed—forever.

Inspiration Suggestions

> *Faith isn't faith until it's all you're holding on to. Unknown*

> *Never be afraid to trust an unknown future to a known God. Corrie Ten Boom*

> *Don't ask God to guide your steps if you're not willing to move your feet. Unknown*

> *I have learned that faith means trusting in advance what will only make sense in reverse. Philip Yancey*

> *Then call on me when you are in trouble, and I will rescue you, and you will give me glory." Psalm 50:15*

> *God is our refuge and strength, always ready to help in times of trouble. Psalm 46:1*

> *Though I am surrounded by troubles, you will protect me from the*

anger of my enemies. You reach out your hand, and the power of your right hand saves me. Psalm 138:7

➢ *Song – "Jesus, Friend of Sinners" by Casting Crowns**

  Song – "Even If" by MercyMe*

➢ *Song – "Eye of the Storm" by Ryan Stevenson **

*Video available at https://bit.ly/2I38TXv

Reflect

1. How often do you feel lonely?

2. Do you ever feel like God is far away or that he has deserted you?

3. Have you ever been knocked down by one of life's storms and wondered where to turn for help? What did you do?

4. Have you ever wanted the hurt to stop but didn't know where to turn? What did you do?

5. Have you ever wanted to run away from your problems? What did you do?

6. If you answered yes to any of the last three questions and you're still reading this book, I assume whatever you did didn't help. Have you tried turning to God for help? Why not?

7. What would it look like in your life if you started trusting God with your problems? What would you need to start doing? What would you need to stop doing?

8. Which Inspiration Suggestions did you choose to explore, and which stood out you'd like to remember?

9. What action steps do you need to take to implement what you've discovered in this chapter?

7

I Need to Ask Those Who Know

Finding Professional Support

If I hear one more person say, "Just think happy thoughts," I think I'll explode out of frustration.

It's not about being happy or sad.

It's not about being stressed or overwhelmed.

I didn't just have a bad day.

What I'm feeling and experiencing isn't normal! Why can't people understand that?

Depression or Sadness

Nothing strikes fear in the average person more than a diagnosis of Ebola. It instills an immediate need to steer clear of anyone infected with this disease. Unfortunately, that's the reaction you often receive when you tell people you have a mental illness.

There's a stigma that accompanies the diagnosis of mental illness, causing many people to shy away from you. It's not for fear of catching the disease, as with Ebola, but out of fear of the unknown. Are you fragile? Can you manage the stress and anxiety of the situation? Will you "go crazy" without warning?

While some lean towards the Ebola response, avoiding you at all cost, that's only because they've confused depression with sadness. Many people think depression is just an extreme version of sadness. However, I can assure you, they are worlds apart. At least that's my experience.

Let's look at the difference between a cold and the flu, for instance. While they are both medical conditions, I think their differences most clearly make my point.

When you see the doctor, he diagnoses you with a cold and tells you to go home and get some rest. A hot bowl of chicken soup and an entire box of tissues, and you start to feel like yourself again after seven to ten stuffy-headed, sleepless nights.

What about when he diagnoses you with the flu? He'll write you a prescription, which will take an irritating eternity to fill at the pharmacy, and send you home to get some rest.

The symptoms of a cold and the flu are very similar, yet they are quite different. With one, you generally get better on your own, while the other requires medical intervention to resolve.

Sadness and depression resemble the cold and flu. They look very similar. Many of the symptoms are the same. However, one generally gets better on its own, while the other requires medical attention.

Depression, like other mental illnesses, will not get better on its own. It requires medical intervention. Unfortunately, the negative stigma attached to receiving professional help for depression means it's not uncommon for it to go untreated. I'm a perfect example of allowing my mental illness to go untreated.

You might not seek the help of a doctor, but you *will* get unsolicited help from everyone else. When you have a physical illness, family members, neighbors, coworkers, and friends don't typically offer to treat you. But when you have a mental illness, they often chime in with advice. They want to help treat your symptoms and make you feel better. If it were only that simple. No chicken soup on the planet will make your depression go away.

Cigna Well Aware for Better Health© says:

> Feeling depressed has become a common way for people to describe the feelings they have when they experience stress, frustration, or sadness. These feelings are a normal reaction to events or situations that are upsetting, frustrating, stressful or

difficult. However, they are different from depression.[1]

To make matters worse, when it comes to mental health issues, there's no one right answer or perfect treatment that always works on every person. Some may be able to simply change their diet and start exercising to manage their symptoms, while others need hospitalization, therapy, medication, and other interventions to manage theirs.

Each medical professional in the mental health field has different skills and abilities when it comes to the treatment of depression. Just as Paul tells us in Romans 12:4-5, "Each has a different gift which works together to serve God," each medical practitioner approaches depression with the skills they've been given, which work together to serve your medical needs.

My Recovery Journey

My family doctor was the first stop on my long road to recovery. Unfortunately, many hours spent waiting at the doctor's office only landed me in the lab. I walked out of there with a pin-cushioned arm that turned into colorful bruising over the next few days. Follow that up with another visit to the doctor's office for results that showed nothing, and my blood began to boil.

I didn't want them to find anything catastrophic, but I certainly wanted them to find something, anything, that would explain what I was experiencing. My sick day balance went down, along with my bank balance, with nothing to show for either.

For many people, a deficiency in some chemical will show up on the lab work, and suddenly—problem solved. Not the case for me. Repeated annual check-ups and routine blood work never revealed any quick medical fix for me. On I walked with the feeling something just wasn't right. *(NOTE: While I make light of this experience, it's always advisable to get an annual check-up and have routine blood work taken to detect problems early.)*

Without answers, I trudged on, wondering where I should go next. I kept telling myself that only the rich have therapists and only the weird pay someone to listen to them. Yet, both are incorrect and minimize the work of professional Licensed Mental Health Counselors and psychologists.

While what they do is often referred to as talk therapy, these professionals do more than listen to you talk. They help you cope with difficult situations in your life as well as assist in processing your thoughts and feelings. They help make sense of the chaos.

My admission of rape there in the church lobby is what landed me in my first psychologist's office. I was advised to see a professional to help me talk about the difficult issue I was finally facing. I suppose the referral was appropriate, since I exhibited no signs of depression at the time. Why? Because I had ignored the issue for twenty years. In my pastor's mind, I wasn't depressed or mentally ill, I just needed to talk through my past problems and how they might have affected my life.

I can't fault him for that. After all, I didn't look mentally ill. I didn't act mentally ill. But the truth of the matter is, I was mentally ill. While psychotherapy/talk therapy is a critical piece of dealing with depression, many times it can't stand alone. However, as with the medical evaluation, it's a good place to start.

Talking helped for periods of time, but I would always return to the feeling that something wasn't right. I needed more. I was one of those people who refused to admit a psychiatrist might help them, because in order for that to happen, I would have had to admit I had a problem—I was mentally ill.

Was is the operative word in that sentence. I've come a long way since then in my understanding of mental illness. Now, as an experienced and educated mental health sufferer, I can easily say, "Hi, my name is Vicki, and I have a mental illness."

It took forty years, but I can finally admit I was powerless over my disease and my life had become unmanageable. That admission was the first step to getting the help I needed.

However, my first visit with a psychiatrist in search of medication to help with my illness came long after that shocking admission in the church lobby. I had gone in and out of psychologist's offices for talk therapy through the years never quite finding one I felt made a difference.

Breakdown #1

That all changed after my first breakdown, when I was hospitalized in the psychiatric ward of the local hospital. Not an experience I can recommend. I was already traumatized by the rape. Facing the trauma twenty years later and realizing the negative effects on my life only magnified my pain.

As I waited to be checked in, after being direct-admitted by my family doctor, I remember a brief visit by my pastor. I remember the anguish on his face as he pleaded with me to tell them I wouldn't hurt myself. "They'll keep you here," he pleaded, as if staying in this place was worse than any fate he could imagine. I quickly found out why.

The nurse led me to a private room where they conducted a thorough search to ensure I wasn't concealing anything I might use to hurt myself. Humiliating! They then rifled through my clothing before returning it to me minus my shoelaces, watch, and jewelry. I was then escorted by the arm through a set of double doors, which sounded like a vault opening. The sounds of people crying, talking loudly, and shuffling in and out came from what I later learned was the day room.

Again, escorted by the arm as if a prisoner, I was led to my room about halfway down the hall. I was given a small bag of toiletries and given a set of rules. I'll be honest; I don't remember much about what was said because a panic attack seized me as I stared wide-eyed at the very large man directly across the hall, who glared back at me. I remember thinking, "He's crazy. He's going to hurt me. I'm not crazy. Why am I here? I AM NOT CRAZY."

After a cold, sleepless night huddled against the wall with my pillow in front of me for protection and a supervised shower the next morning, I finally met with a doctor. He introduced himself, and the floodgate holding back all the fear and emotion I had locked inside me over the previous twenty-four hours burst open. I cried and pleaded for help. This was my first encounter with a psychiatrist. Not the best!

In order to be released, I had to agree to see a psychiatrist regularly and maintain a strict medication schedule. Of course, I would've agreed to anything at that point. I wasn't crazy, but if I stayed in that place any longer, I would've been.

Fast-forward past almost two decades of monthly psychiatrist and psychologist appointments, three or four unsuccessful medications, and periods with the appearance of mental health, and then we land in 2014.

More specifically, October 29, 2014.

Breakdown #2

As I sat in a heap of tears in my psychiatrist's office that day, she told my husband I needed to be hospitalized. I flew into a frenzy of protests, visualizing my previous horrifying experience. Fortunately, this doctor knew me, and I trusted her. She had helped me find a medication that seemed to help, and she shared my Christian beliefs. She knew my background, and she cared enough to have a plan that suited my specific needs and insecurities. She announced I would be going to a behavioral hospital about an hour from my home and assured me this place was the right place for me. I trusted her so, cautiously, I agreed.

After a quick stop at the house to gather a few things, my husband drove me to the hospital and quietly parked the car. I sat frozen in my seat. He walked around, opened the door, and gently took my arm to help me from the car. He silently, but tenderly, wrapped his arm around my waist and gently pressed me forward towards the door. Without a word, we entered the calm, brightly lit lobby. My husband informed the receptionist about our issue, and she kindly informed us to have a seat to await the next available intake counselor.

A caring young man greeted us and asked us to follow him to a small office where we completed the intake process. Once completed, he suggested he'd wait outside while I said good-bye to my husband. We shared a long, tearful embrace that would have crushed an elephant, followed by a whispered *I love you*; and then, he was gone.

The intake counselor returned with a smile of compassion and offered to show me to my room in what he affectionately referred to as the penthouse suite. He led me through a set of doors (locked, of course) out into a beautiful courtyard filled with grass, trees, and picnic tables, where I saw people who seemed to be enjoying themselves in the sun as if on vacation. There was an eerie silence. It was peaceful.

I noticed the wrought iron fence surrounding the courtyard, but it didn't evoke a sense of panic as I might have expected. He waved his badge in front of a sensor at the next building and opened the door for me to enter. There were people moving around in the hallway; others sat quietly in their rooms. Some light, cheerful conversation at the end of the hall made its way to me. No commotion, loud noises, or tension.

He led me to the third door on the left and allowed me to enter the room quietly on my own. He compassionately wished me well and disappeared down the hall. There in that quiet room off the hallway I shared with twelve other penthouse guests, I spent the next eleven days.

Then I was released into what they refer to as the partial hospitalization program. You continue to be in therapy sessions all day, visit with the psychiatrist, and eat meals as a group, but you're allowed to go home overnight. My husband managed my medications for me, as I was still very unsure of myself and more than a little afraid of… basically everything. While I felt a sense of freedom in this outpatient program, I spent most of my evenings in my room alone.

Nine days later, I was released. I was paralyzed with fear and doubt, and my husband once again gently nudged me forward through the parking lot, this time towards the car that would take me on my final trip home.

Was this the beginning or the end?

Could I actually do it on my own?

I had no idea. I only knew I'd learned to depend on God for every breath, every thought, and every step I took during those twenty days. There was no way I could stop depending on him now. Armed with the coping strategies learned in group therapy and from my Bible, I determined I would not only survive but succeed at this thing called life with a mental illness.

I eventually discovered it was a beginning and an end. The answer was yes, I could actually survive. But not alone! God checked out of that hospital with me and has been by my side ever since.

My recovery journey is just that—*my* journey. Your recovery will inevitably be different; everyone's is. As you look at my journey, don't be discouraged by the early negative experiences I shared. When the timing was right, and I was ready to admit I needed help and I couldn't go on without it, I was able to make a connection with a doctor who understood me and knew how to best get me the help I needed. These factors combined with an intimate walk with God made all the difference in my later experience and the outcome.

Mental Health Professionals

In the last chapter, I provided a cheat sheet to help you develop your own intimate walk with God. Here, let me provide a cheat sheet outlining each of the medical professionals I encountered along my journey. Remember, different people connect in different ways. Don't be afraid to keep searching for the right medical professional until you find someone with whom you share a deep connection.

General Practitioner	Your family doctor provides general medical care. She can identify and treat any general

	medical issues that may explain your symptoms. Make sure to have annual check-ups and routine bloodwork to increase your chances of catching any health concerns early. If your doctor doesn't take the time to understand your concerns and answer your questions, keep looking.
Psychiatrists Psychiatric Wards Psychiatric Hospitals	**Psychiatrists** are medical doctors who specialize in the treatment of psychiatric, or mental health, disorders. As an MD, they can prescribe medication. For me, medication was necessary. I've had a couple of times where my dosage, or medication choice, wasn't meeting my physical needs. As soon as we fixed the medication issue, I was better able to manage my symptoms. **Psychiatric wards** are special wings in your local hospital, while a **psychiatric hospital** is a stand-alone facility. Both are designed specifically for the treatment of serious mental health disorders.
Mental Health Counselors Psychologists	Psychotherapy, also known as talk therapy, provides an opportunity for you to have an outside, objective third party help you process what you're feeling, thinking, and doing. A common form of talk therapy is Cognitive Behavioral Therapy (CBT). Cognitive has to do with your brain or thoughts. Behavior has to do with your actions. CBT helps you see the relationship between your thoughts and your actions. Unfortunately for me, my brain knew what I needed to do long before my actions caught up. I still struggle with some specific things, but I've found an entirely empowering connection between my thoughts and my reactions that has helped me change many destructive behavior patterns.
Mental Health	While technically a psychiatric hospital, these

Hospitals Behavioral Hospitals	facilities focus on empowering a patient towards independent self-care. They're not long-term solutions. As you saw from my experience, the compassion, sincerity, and respect I received was a critical factor in feeling safe enough to finally let go and admit I needed help.
Insurance Provider	My insurance provider, Cigna, goes to great lengths to assist with long-term self-care in patients with various ailments, including depression. Through their Well Aware for Better Health© program, they provided me with the following services: self-assessments, wellness coaching, online coaching, depression toolkit, and *Your Depression Workbook*.[2] Check with your provider for similar services.

Everyone needs different levels of help. Through the years, I had treated the most obvious symptoms with medication and occasional talk therapy and got back to work. I never had the time to look further or try to figure out what was wrong. Let me rephrase that—I never took the time.

Treat the Cause, Not Just the Symptoms

You can treat the symptoms of a heart attack with pain killers and anti-anxiety medications. However, unless you look further, unless you take the time to see what's causing those symptoms, nothing will change. Your disease will continue to progress. The unseen and untreated damage going on inside your body will eventually kill you.

Just like pain killers won't cure a heart attack, thinking happy thoughts won't cure depression. Take the time, *make* the time, to find the right people, and care enough about yourself to get help. Start with your family doctor if you don't know where else to start. Just start! People won't have to tell you to think happy thoughts once you start successfully managing and treating your depression.

My experiences prove the old Buddhist proverb that says, "When the student is ready, the teacher will appear." I believe that's the theme of the parables Jesus used to teach the Pharisees. In Luke 18:9-14, Jesus tells a tale of two men entering the temple to pray. One makes a show of his prayers, while the other humbles himself before God, recognizing his place as a sinner. Jesus declares the righteous, showy man would be humbled while the humbled man would become righteous.

How does this particular parable relate to my story? I was that self-righteous, showy man. I craved the love, respect, and attention of men. However, I now strive to be the humbled man recognizing my place as a sinner. I've read this verse multiple times throughout my life. But only after this experience did I finally understand it. I was finally ready, and God, my teacher, appeared.

Inspiration Suggestions

➢ *Having a mental disorder isn't easy, and it's even harder when people assume you can just get over it. Unknown*

➢ *The only thing more exhausting than having a mental illness is pretending like you don't. Unknown*

➢ *Promise me you'll always remember—you're braver than you believe, and stronger than you seem, and smarter than you think. Christopher Robin*

➢ *If there is no struggle, there is no progress. Fredrick Douglas*

➢ *Start by doing what's necessary, then do what's possible; and suddenly you are doing the impossible. Saint Francis of Assisi*

➢ *Mental pain is less dramatic than physical pain, but it is more common and also harder to bear. The frequent attempt to conceal mental pain increases the burden: It is easier to say, "My tooth is aching" than to say, "My heart is broken." C. S. Lewis*

➢ *Your present circumstances don't determine where you can go; they merely determine where you start. Nido Qubein*

➢ *Song – "I Am Not Alone" by Kari Jobe**

➢ *Song – "Sparrows" by Jason Gray**

➢ *Song – "Never Too Far Gone" by Jordan Feliz**

*Video available at https://bit.ly/2I38TXv

Reflect

1. Have you seen your family doctor recently and discussed your symptoms? Have you had blood work done to determine if there is a chemical or hormonal cause for your symptoms?

2. Have you seen a psychologist or therapist recently? If not, what's stopping you?

3. If you've seen a psychologist or therapist, did you feel a connection with them after a few visits? If not, what's stopping you from trying to find another that might be a better fit?

4. Have you seen a psychiatrist recently? Are you taking medication if prescribed? Are you experiencing side effects? Have you discussed whether there are better options available?

5. Have you ever been hospitalized for your mental illness? Was it a positive or negative experience? Have you discussed it with your psychiatrist for future reference?

6. Have you fully committed to getting better, or are you simply treating the symptoms?

7. Have you taken the time to get to the root cause of your depression, or are you continually pushing it under the radar because it's too inconvenient or expensive to deal with it?

8. Which Inspiration Suggestions did you choose to explore, and which stood out you'd like to remember?

9. What action steps do you need to take to implement what you've discovered in this chapter?

8

I Need to Accept Help

Leaning on Your Support System

Some men would rather die than ask for directions. My husband and father both fall into this category. Thank goodness for the invention of GPS. In a similar display of stubbornness, many teenagers would rather crash and burn on a test than admit in a classroom full of their peers they don't know how to do something. Women do it too. We'd rather work ourselves into exhaustion and despair than admit we can't manage all the tasks we take on as working moms with active families.

Nobody likes to admit they need help. Nobody wants to be a burden, and it's never fun to feel unable to manage what others seemingly do with ease. However, no one came out of the womb able to function independently.

Every adult on this planet needed help with basic life-sustaining needs such as food, shelter, and safety as a child. At what point did it become "uncool" to ask for help. I'd have to say somewhere around the preteen years, but any parent of a two-year old will tell you the quest for independence starts there.

Whether it be at two, twelve, or twenty, this need for independence, and to prove we don't need anybody's help, is the beginning of our downfall. We've all needed help at one time or another. So why is it so hard to say those two simple words—help me?

Asking For and Receiving Help

A couple of years ago, our best friend's son was diagnosed with a blood disease that required a bone marrow transplant. What was supposed to be a 30-day hospital stay turned into almost 300 days, with several of those being "we don't think he's going to make it" kind of days.

Whether it be at two, twelve, or twenty, this need for independence, and to prove we don't need anybody's help, is the beginning of our downfall. We've all needed help at one time or another. So why is it so hard to say those two simple words—help me?

As you can imagine, they needed help to get through that difficult time. They needed a shoulder to cry on, financial support to pay bills, someone to listen to them pour out their greatest fears, someone to drive their other son to and from school and the hospital an hour away. They needed a person, another human being, who could actually be there with them at a time when they didn't feel that God heard or cared about what was happening to their child.

One of my very close coworkers knew about the struggle and the support we'd been providing to this family. One day, I commented about taking dinner to another church friend who'd just been released from the hospital following surgery. My coworker said, "Wow! You have a lot of needy people at your church." I stood in her doorway pondering that for a minute. Then I said, "Not really; we just have a lot of people willing to ask for help when they need it."

The interesting thing about that is, I was not one of those people. I realized after my breakdown that I hadn't asked for help because I wasn't willing to ask for help. I'd compared my need against the need of others and decided God would probably focus on real problems, not trivial ones like mine.

The problem with this mindset is that depression isn't a trivial problem. Depression is a disease. Just like any other disease, when you need help, you should ask for it. This is a lesson I learned too late to avoid my breakdown, but it was a valuable lesson, nonetheless. One I've finally learned to implement during difficult times.

When I'm struggling emotionally, or feel myself sliding into a downward spiral, I ask for prayer support. When I need a shoulder to cry on, I ask someone to come sit with me. When I need time alone to recover from a panic attack, or just decompress from what's going on around me, I ask my husband and others to keep an eye on me, so I don't allow that alone time to become a habit.

Everyone Needs Help – Caring for One Another

In 1 Corinthians 12:25-27, we're reminded we're all part of Christ's body. We each have a different role to play. When one part of the body suffers, we all suffer. When one part rejoices, we all rejoice. In the Amplified Bible, verse 25 says, "...but the members all alike should have a mutual interest in and care for one another." We were put on this earth to care for one another.

It's so easy to forget the many blessings I have when something is overwhelming me. Fortunately, God doesn't rank needs and decide one is worthier of his attention than another. God loves every one of us and provides help in different ways, and at different levels, to meet our individual needs.

Sometimes we need to be the one to ask for help. It's hard. Believe me; I know. That ugly sin, pride, raises its head often in my life. When it does, I need to put it aside and just ask for help. When others see I'm struggling and offer to help, I no longer turn them away. God has called them to care for me. Likewise, I believe he has called me to swallow my pride and let them.

Everyone needs help with something. Some more than others. I've needed help many times throughout my life. Ok, I'll be honest. I've needed help several times just this week. While my needs this week are trivial in the whole scheme of things, I have several friends at this very moment who are struggling with their own life-threatening illness or have a family member who's struggling.

It's so easy to forget the many blessings I have when something is overwhelming me. Fortunately, God doesn't rank needs and decide one is worthier of his attention than another. God loves every one of us and provides help in different ways, and at different levels, to meet our individual needs.

My need for help this week has been emotional support, whereas my friend needed help at a moment of crisis in the treatment of her child's life-threatening disease. If I fall into the comparison trap, I might believe God is too busy helping my friend and her child to have time to help me. Fortunately for me, that's not how God works. We both have needs, and God desires to meet all our needs, no matter how big or small.

God saw early on in his creation that man needed help. He said, "It is not good for man to be alone. I will send him a helper." (Genesis 2:18) I outlined in chapter six the many ways I can be assured God is always with me. He's not only with me, he desires to help me and is more than able to do so.

But as the creation story points out, sometimes God sends other people to help me. Why? Because sometimes I just need a good hug. God understands that.

While God already sent all his believers a helper, comforter, counselor, advocate, intercessor, and strengthener in the Holy Spirit (John 16:7), I still need someone to hold me when I cry and to care for me when I'm sick. God provides others he's placed around me to fill that role in my life. In the same way, I've been placed around others to fill that role for them.

A Life Verse from God

At a particularly difficult time in my life, God gave me what I call my life verse. It's 1 Peter 5:6-11. It reminds me to humble myself and admit I can't do things on my own. If I do that, God will lift me up when his timing is right.

It reminds me God is always looking out for me and wants to help me if I'll give him my problems.

It cautions me to always be on the lookout for the enemy who wants to destroy me. Just as animals encircle their young or wounded when under attack by a predator, I have a protective circle of family and friends who will do the same for me. Sometimes, I need to be on the inside of that protective circle. I need to allow others to protect and care for me during difficult times. However, others are struggling and under attack as well, so sometimes I'll need to be on the outside of that protective circle. That's my turn to protect and care for them.

Finally, it gives me the reassurance that while I may be suffering now, it won't last forever. God loves me, so when the time is right, he personally will come pick me up, set me firmly in place, and make me stronger than ever before.

Just Be There

God has placed people around us to care for us and protect us; but sometimes, when I'm struggling, I just want to be left alone. I don't want to be around people because I'm afraid they'll judge me, look down on me, think I'm weak, or worse yet, think I'm a whiner.

No one likes to be alone. But in the mind of someone struggling with depression, it's better to be alone than to be judged. I often felt if I looked fine, people would believe I was fine. If they saw me suffering they would feel pity for me. As long as they couldn't see me suffering, they'd love and respect me.

I remember when my husband came to visit me the day after I was admitted to the hospital. When I was escorted into the family visiting lounge, he walked over, put his arms around me, held me tight, and said, "I love you." After a long, quiet embrace, I pulled away and softly asked, "Why?"

He just stood and stared at me as if I'd asked him to explain the origin of the universe. It seemed like an eternity before he answered. He stood frozen in time perplexed by my lack of expected response to his profession of love. I remember thinking, in what was most likely only a split-second pause, that he loved me because he had to love me. After all, he'd promised before God and many witnesses to love me in sickness and in health. He didn't really love me. I thought that he'd rather be anywhere but standing in that visiting room taking care of his helpless wife. I remember feeling pitiful.

I collapsed onto the floor and pulled my knees tight into my chest, dropped my head onto my knees, and began to cry. His response made me realize that, although I felt pitiful, he definitely didn't pity me. He genuinely loved me.

He slowly lowered himself to the chair behind me and pulled me close, straddling my balled-up heap of hurt on the floor. Then he bent over me and just held me in his arms with his head resting on top of mine. We sat there, speechless.

In the moments that followed, he didn't need to speak. His tender act of love spoke volumes. Suddenly, all these little things in our marriage that had annoyed me for years seemed insignificant. All the times I tried things and failed, nagged at him about his annoying habits, and complained about our situation didn't matter. The only thing that mattered was the fact he'd always loved me. And somehow, he still did.

I don't know if he ever actually answered my question regarding why he loved me; I just know there was no longer a need for him to do so. He understood the only thing he could do at that moment was reassure me of his love, hold me, and be present in the moment. He could meet me where I was and hold my hand while I got to where I wanted to be, even if neither of us could see where that might be. He continued to show up in that visiting room day after day and just be there, just be present in my life.

At that point, I had nothing to offer him, or anyone, in exchange for those acts of kindness. I was, by necessity, completely focused on getting better. It required great patience on his part to continue to just show up and hold me, reassure me, and love me until I was capable of asking and accepting other help. Yet still, he came.

Find Someone Who's Already Been There

I'm not the first person to suffer from depression. Neither are you. When I finally reached the point where I could ask for help from others, I knew I needed to find someone who'd been there before. I needed someone who'd understand where I'd been and the issues I was facing daily.

Many, if not all, of the twelve-step programs, such as Alcoholics Anonymous and Co-Dependents Anonymous, are based on having a sponsor to walk with you. A sponsor is someone who has walked in your shoes, has overcome their own struggle, and is now available any time day or night to help you on your journey.

While the phrase "it takes one to know one" is often seen as a quick retort to an insult hurled by someone else, for the purposes of these recovery programs, it means something entirely different. An alcoholic can spot another alcoholic from a great distance. A drug user can do the same. Why? Because they've been there. They know the signs, symptoms, behaviors, and excuses.

The same holds true for any person facing a diagnosis of depression. If you want to overcome an addiction, you find someone who's already overcome that addiction. In order to overcome depression, you need to look for someone who's overcome depression, someone who's already been where you are now and survived it.

One of the songs that compelled me to write my story was "The Words I Would Say" by Sidewalk Prophets. The lyrics caused me to ponder what I'd want to say to someone getting ready to go somewhere I'd already been—through depression.

I'd want to give them hope for the future. I'd want to be present with them in whatever moment they were in, just as my husband met me where I was. This person isn't necessarily a professional, like the ones I mentioned earlier. While these professionals are essential to your recovery, you also need someone who may not have a fancy certificate or degree, but who does have firsthand life experience. This person is an invaluable member of your support team.

There are many Twelve Step© programs out there whose sole purpose is to support those experiencing difficulty in their lives by providing a support system of understanding people who've already walked in those shoes. The same concept will work for you. Find an accountability partner or sponsor to walk with you on your journey.

You Are Only Alone If You Choose to Be

As a teenager, I remember singing songs into my hairbrush microphone about friends standing by friends in a time of need. Songs about always having someone you could go to for help. Two that stick in my mind still today, decades later, are "You've Got a Friend" and "Lean on Me." Both share the idea friends and loved ones are waiting in the wings to be there for us in our time of need. I could easily recite those lyrics from memory back then (still can, actually), so why then didn't I call out for help? Why didn't I tell someone about my rape?

My older sister and I were very close growing up. We did almost everything together and I looked up to her. I knew I could tell her anything and she would listen. I knew I could do anything, and she would help me. One year, in high school, we were both cast to perform in the school musical *Carousel*. A key theme in that musical was the feeling of loneliness and despair.

A song from that musical blossomed into a song of triumph still sung today, "You'll Never Walk Alone." I knew as long as my sister was there with me, I'd never walk alone. However, as close as we were, I couldn't even tell her about the rape. I couldn't tell her about my struggle. I chose to walk alone. I shut God out, and I shut my sister out.

Thirteen years later, my sister died unexpectedly from a brain aneurism. I felt like a part of me died with her. As teenagers do, we had made different choices in life and started running with different friends. Eventually we got married, started families, and drifted apart somewhat as people do when their lives become busy with new things. Still, we were linked by an unspoken commitment to always be there. Only now, she wasn't.

I'd been there for her through the years. She'd never hesitated to call on me when something was wrong, I'd always drop everything to help. She trusted me and leaned on that bond we had. I hadn't. Why?

That question still bothers me today. I suppose it was because I was afraid. I was afraid if she knew the truth, she'd no longer love me and no longer be there for me. That's an agonizing admission of the truth. I chose to be alone rather than trust someone.

I dream sometimes about how my life might've been different if I had trusted her. If I had trusted someone. Anyone. One day, as I walked through a craft fair, I saw the lyrics to "You'll Never Walk Alone" on a small framed art piece. I bought it and kept it close for many years, always thinking of her. I've now passed it on to my son, a Liverpool Football Club fanatic who sings it from the bottom of his heart, and the top of his lungs, at the beginning of every game.

I wonder if he sees me in those words, the way I saw my sister in them. Will he ever turn to me in a time of need? If a time arises, will he trust me enough with his pain? I can only hope so.

Sometimes we choose to be alone. Sometimes we need to get away. We need to process and ponder what's going on. However, as there are times and seasons for everything, you shouldn't always be alone. Actually, let me rephrase that. You should never be alone. There's no need for it. Someone loves you as much as my sister loved me. Infinitely more than that, actually. Swallow your pride. Reach out. Say those two simple words—help me!

Inspiration Suggestions

➢ *Sometimes the only answer people are looking for when they ask for help is that they won't have to face the problem alone. Mark Amend*

➢ *Asking for help isn't weak; it's a great example of how to take care of yourself. Charlie Brown*

> *Healing takes time and asking for help is a courageous first step. Mariska Hargitay*

> *Sometimes in life, you can fall down holes you can't climb out of by yourself. That's what friends and family are for—to help. They can't help, however, unless you let them know you're down there. Meg Cabot*

> *The best advice I can give to anyone going through a rough patch is to never be afraid to ask for help. Demi Lovato*

> *I am a strong person, but every now and then I also need someone to take my hand and say everything will be alright. Unknown*

> *Song – "Lean on Me" by Bill Withers**

> *Song – "You've Got a Friend" by Carole King**

> *Song – "You'll Never Walk Alone" by Richard Rodgers and Oscar Hammerstein**

*Video available at https://bit.ly/2I38TXv

Reflect

1. Do you avoid asking for help? What can you do to change that?

2. What's currently going on in your life that might be easier to handle if someone were able to help support you emotionally?

3. What would be the best way for them to support you (prayer, finances, someone to listen, to be there for you, keep an eye on you)?

4. Who might you ask to provide that support?

5. Does pride stop you from asking for help? What are you afraid might happen? What could happen if you push past your fear and ask anyway?

6. Have you ever compared your need for help with someone else's and decided your need was too small to warrant help?

7. Has God given you a life verse, a verse you hold dear in your heart, for times when you struggle? What is it? How does it help you?

8. Who might be a good accountability partner for you?

9. Which Inspiration Suggestions did you choose to explore, and which stood out you'd like to remember?

10. What action steps do you need to take to implement what you've discovered in this chapter?

PART
III

How Do I Get Better?

9

I Need to See Things Differently

Perspective

You have one minute to write ten words to describe yourself positively.

Ready, set, go!

That was my task according to the group therapy leader. I spent the first thirty seconds just staring at the paper with complete paralysis. Then it hit me. I'm kind! That was easy. I'm on a roll now. Words will just flow out like someone turned on the faucet. Then … nothing.

Time's up. Put your pencils down. Now, count 'em up. Did you get ten? Uh… NO. I got one. One positive word to describe me. At least it was a good word, right? It's good to be kind, isn't it?

Now, turn your paper over. In one minute, write ten words to positively describe your parent, spouse, child, or a close friend. Ready, set, go!

I got this one. My children are kind and compassionate. They're smart, generous, witty … and the list went on.

Time's up. Put your pencils down. Once again, I counted. This time I not only had ten, I had more. Why was there such a discrepancy? Why did I have such a hard time seeing the good in myself, but such an easy time seeing it in others?

Self-Hatred

In my case, the answer to that question is called self-hatred. From the moment that fourteen-year-old girl judged herself by the actions of others, I've hated myself. I hated how I felt, how I looked, how I acted in the following years, and how I failed to act on my own behalf. I hated how I felt weak and unlovable. I hated having others look down on me. I hated feeling as if what I wanted didn't matter, what made me happy was irrelevant. I lived for the sole purpose of making others happy. While putting others first is a noble gesture, it was a necessity for me at that point, not a choice.

Forty years later, I was still judging myself by the feelings and actions of others, or at least my perception of those feelings and actions. If I couldn't make them happy, I felt unlovable. If I made a simple mistake, I felt unworthy. I've learned through decades of living on a self-imposed merit-based system to focus on all my failures. To focus on my unworthiness.

Although I went through periods where my faith was strong, and I truly believed God loved me, more often than not, I felt I'd gone too far to be forgiven. Therefore, I'd gone too far to be loved. It was just too hard to understand how I could mess up so badly and still be loved. My shame and guilt overwhelmed my understanding of grace.

Your Mind May Be Your Biggest Bully

Fortunately, in God's eyes, my past and current actions are not a measure of who I am or what I'm worth to him. My actions don't determine whether I'm good or bad. Bad choices and bad actions don't make me a bad person. They make me human.

As a human, it's the focus of my heart that determines my worth. As a Christian, the focus of my heart is to love God and accept the sacrifice he made just so he could spend eternity with me. That God would sacrifice his son for me is a hard thing to believe, but it's true. He loved me that much and wanted to spend eternity with me.

Bad choices and bad actions don't make me a bad person. They make me human.

Over the years, I'd come to believe God was like human men and only loved me when I was doing things to make him happy. Nothing could be farther from the truth. God loves me because I'm his. Even now while I'm still sinning, God loves me. (Romans 5:8)

Someone once told me we should never allow the self-hatred we feel to control us, to bully us. As an educator, I know all about bullies. Just as I would never allow a bully to hurt someone physically with their actions, I also would never allow them to use their words to hurt someone emotionally. I'd stand up to that bully in a heartbeat and put an end to his attacks. Yet I allow the negative words and feelings inside my mind to hurt me every day. How is that any different? It's time for that to stop. It's time to stand up to that bully inside my head and end his attacks against me.

Bullies Steal Hope and Joy

Peter probably dealt with attacks from his own bully after denying any knowledge of Jesus following his arrest. After all, Peter had great hope for a future with Jesus as his people's leader. He had hope for the kingdom of heaven Jesus promised. But those hopes had just been ripped from him as he watched Jesus taken away by the soldiers.

I allow the negative words and feelings inside my mind to hurt me every day. How is that any different? It's time for that to stop. It's time to stand up to that bully inside my head and end his attacks against me.

Then the questions came. Was that you I saw with Jesus? Aren't you one of his followers? Three times he denied knowing Jesus. I suspect Peter justified the denials as necessary to save his own life. Still, he'd given up everything to follow Jesus. And now, Jesus was gone. Just like that, Peter's hope for the future was gone. I know that feeling of having all hope for the future ripped from you, so I understand the desperation Peter must have felt.

Each time the question came, Peter had to make a decision—acknowledge Jesus and face sure death or deny any knowledge of him and live. Three times, he faced that decision, and three times he gave the same answer. The decision seemed simple—live or die. The government was planning to execute Jesus. Anyone who was with him was also sure to be killed.

Without Jesus, their leader, the promised kingdom was gone. The disciples had nothing left. There was no point in losing their lives along with their hopes and dreams. Peter wanted to live, so he made the only choice he felt like he could—he denied Jesus. He did what he thought he had to do to survive. He left Jesus behind, along with his hopes and dreams, and tried to move on with his life. Alone.

I understand that choice. I made the same one.

I'm sure Peter's head was filled with regret about his decision the minute he heard the rooster crow. Then the never-ending questions overtook his thoughts. Would things have been different if he'd acknowledged Jesus for who he was? Would he have been able to convince the rulers to spare the life of Jesus? Could he have saved the ministry they'd worked so hard to build? How could he have done something so terrible?

That is where the self-hatred most likely began. Not only was Jesus dead, but Peter couldn't help but think what a horrible person he must be. He had lied about knowing Jesus just to save himself. How could he live with himself?

The hours and days between the crucifixion and resurrection must have been agonizing for him. What would happen to him? Not only was he in physical danger from the Pharisees but he must have had agonizing mental anguish thinking about what had happened and what was ahead for him. How had things gone so terribly wrong?

Just like Peter, I also had incredible hope for the future, and in an instant, I watched it all slip away. After it was over, as I cowered alone and afraid, I too had to make a decision. Live or die? My decision wasn't a physical life or death choice like Peter's, but it certainly felt that way. I also left Jesus behind, along with all my hopes and dreams, and tried to move on with my life. Alone.

Someone Does Understand

I was so overwhelmed by the crisis in my past, I forgot God's promises for my present and my future. In John 16:33, Jesus told us, "The world will make you suffer. But be brave! I have defeated the world!" Jesus suffered too. That's how he understood what Peter went through, and what I went through centuries later. He also understands what you're going through.

From the time Satan was thrown down from heaven to earth there's been a constant struggle for control over my life. Satan wants me to be self-absorbed and broken. He wants me to ignore God's commands for me and do what makes me feel good. He wants to hold me hostage to evil desires.

On the other side of this battle, God wants me to be focused on his love for me, be obedient to his commandments, accept his forgiveness for my sins, and follow in the path he has lovingly set out for me. The battle is real. The war between good and evil rages on.

The Battle's Already Been Won

The battle exists because, although I'm made in God's image, I was also born into a sinful world. However, in 2 Chronicles 20:15 we are assured the battle to defeat evil is not ours, but God's. The battle over my life, and my future, has already been fought and won. Not by me, but by Christ. The price for my life was his life.

That's when Satan lost the right to control me. He's been defeated. I'm assured of that in 1 John 4:3-4. "But, every spirit that does not acknowledge Jesus is not from God. This is the spirit of the antichrist, which you have heard is coming and even now is already in the world. You, dear children, are from God and have overcome them, because the one who is in you is greater than the one who is in the world."

The battle over my life, and my future, has already been fought and won. Not by me, but by Christ. The price for my life was his life.

That doesn't mean Satan will ever stop trying. Until he breathes his last breath on the day of judgment, Satan will do everything within his power to destroy me and try to pull me away from my relationship with God. When that happens, the words of John 16:33 continue to echo in my head, "I have defeated the world."

If that's true, if God's already defeated the evil in our world, it's time to declare victory over evil in my life. Declaring victory is the easy part. Living in that victory, day after day, proves to be the most difficult. But I think that's the point of grace. God's grace is new each morning. He gives me a second chance, a fresh start, every single day.

Who Am I

A fresh start means I can be a new and improved person every day. Tomorrow I can be better than I am today. However, that requires me to know who I am today. Who am I?

Psalm 139:13-14 says I'm fearfully and wonderfully made. What exactly does that mean? I'm not a theologian, but I know it means God took great care to create me with a certain plan or purpose in mind. I am unique. I'm not like any other human being he created. He gave me blue eyes, brown hair, and all the other physical attributes that make me a distinct individual. He gave me a level of intelligence, compassion, and specific talent that make me unique. He then gave me to a middle-class family in the Midwestern part of the United States where I learned to share the interests of other Midwesterners. I love baseball, picnics, family gatherings, and Sunday church services. All these things combined to make me the woman I am today.

Along the way, I had unique experiences that helped mold me into the person I am now. All this leads us to the age-old question—was nature or nurture responsible for who I am? Who I have become? As I said, I'm not a theologian or a scientist, so I can't answer those questions.

What I can say is that I'm certainly a product of my parents' genes; I look like them in many ways. But I'm also very much a product of my environment and the experiences I had along the way. Ultimately, however, I am a child of God (Romans 8:14-15). The Bible tells me I was created in his image (Genesis 1:27). I have his traits and characteristics, and I share his interests and desires. If this is true, and we all were made in his image, how can we all be so different? How can I be unique?

For weeks, my therapist worked with me to define who I am. To determine what made me ... me. She kept telling me, "Before you can learn to love yourself, you have to know who you are and then learn to love those things that make you ... you." Who are you?

I thought that was an easy question. I'm a wife, mother, and lifelong educator. I love reading, exercise, and nature. I'm broken, worthless, and unloved.

She kept telling me those things weren't who I was; those things were what I did and what I felt. She continued to ask, "Who are you?"

Week after week, I pondered what made me unique at the core of my being, only to live in a constant state of frustration with the answers always just out of reach. It's an easy question really; only three simple words, and not even big words. So why couldn't I find the answer?

If wife, mother, and lifelong educator were what I do, and broken, worthless, and unloved were what I felt, then who was I?

Finally, she asked the question in a way that made it all come together. She asked, "What makes you human?" The easy answer is arms, legs, eyes, and ears. But even animals have all those things. Once again, the easy answer didn't work. What made me different from the animals? What made me human? Unique? From that question, came the poem "Who Am I?"

Who Am I?
I am Human – I make mistakes!
I will accept my mistakes as normal and,
I will focus on my successes, not my failures.

I am Human – I have emotions!
I will experience my emotions and,
I will use self-control in order to respond to facts, not feelings!
I am Human – I have a history!
I will accept both good and bad experiences, and
I will cherish my blessings while using what I learned to help others!

I am Human – I have physical flaws!
I will accept what I see in the mirror as a unique creation and,
I will focus on what I can do, instead of what I cannot do.

I am Human – I have strengths and weaknesses!
I will acknowledge I was not made to do everything perfectly and,
I will find ways to use my strengths, while seeking help for my weaknesses.

I am Human – I have unique interests and passions!
I will set aside the expectations of others and,
I will follow my heart, allowing myself to do what brings me joy.

I am Human – I understand right and wrong!
I will do what is right just because it is right and,
I will boldly speak the truth in love to myself, and others, when it is wrong.

I am Human – I am made in the image of God!
I will believe I am a masterpiece and,
I will declare I have a purpose – I am wanted – I am loved!

Vicki L. Huffman, 2015

God knows everything about me (Psalm 139:1-6). He created me with intention, with a plan, and to fulfill a particular purpose within that plan. Just like I might think about vacation plans or financial plans all the time, God thinks about me all the time because I'm a part of his plan. (Psalm 139:17)

He created me with certain traits, so that I would fit into the environment where I was placed. He led me through certain experiences, so I would be able to develop skills and talents to fulfill a very specific role within his plan. And he shared his interests and passions with me in the hopes I would make them my interests and passions too. I am human, yet I am also a child of God.

Becoming a New Person

When I keep my focus squarely on God and his plan for my life, my circumstances tend to fade into the background. The old me was filled with self-hatred that forced me to believe I was still, and always would be, judged for my sin. However, God's Word clearly says, "I am a new creation." That means:

- I'm no longer a slave to sin; I'm a slave to God's perfect plan for my life.

- I'm no longer obligated to follow my fleshly desires; I can choose to follow God's desires.

- I'm no longer sentenced to death for my sins; I have eternal life through Jesus Christ.

- I can be overwhelmed with guilt by my constant inability to keep God's Law or I can live in the knowledge of God's grace.

- I'm no longer restricted to learning about my God through someone else's words; I can learn about him through a daily intimate personal relationship with him.

- I no longer have a desire for wickedness; I desire what is good and holy.

- I can live ashamed of my past and condemned by my thoughts, or I can live as an honorable, forgiven daughter of the God Almighty.

Joshua 24:15 says, "Choose today whom you will serve." When others try to belittle us or question our worth, we need to recognize our worth comes from God, not from anything we have done or will do.

Each day is an opportunity to walk free from the chains of self-hatred. Each day is an opportunity to remember what has been, accept what is, and have joy over what is to come.

Starting Over

In those hours and days following the crucifixion, Peter realized he needed to start over. Everything he thought he knew had changed. Then, in the midst of Peter's turmoil, Jesus appeared to his disciples. Already frightened by what might happen to them, the appearance of Jesus sent the disciples over the top with fear. Jesus asked, "Why are you frightened? Why are your hearts filled with doubt?" (Luke 24:38, NLT) He proceeded to show them the nail marks in his hands and feet, the wound in his side. Suddenly they believed. Once again, they had hope for the future.

When God guides you to the unknown, you have no choice but to trust him.

I've always believed my value came from my ability to make others happy and meet their needs. My breakdown forced me to give up anything that made me feel worthy: my job, my administrative responsibilities at the church, basically, all responsibilities. I could no longer meet anyone's needs, including my own. I was totally dependent on others, and that's the opposite of anything I've ever known or who I've ever been.

When God guides you to the unknown, you have no choice but to trust him. It was only in that moment, when I had nothing else, that I was able to see I actually had everything.

When God is all you have, you quickly discover God was all you ever needed. Only then will you be able to see yourself as God sees you and give up caring what anyone thinks except for him. Only then can you see yourself as a new creation, free of guilt and shame. Only then will you be able to learn how to love yourself. And that's the beginning of hope and joy.

Inspiration Suggestions

➤ *Hate is the byproduct of hurt. Your self-hate is the byproduct of thinking that you have hurt yourself by blowing the chance to get the love you so badly want from others. Teal Swan*

➤ *To establish true self-esteem we must concentrate on our successes and forget about the failures and negatives in our lives. Denis Waitley*

➤ *Don't over-focus on the negatives and under-focus on the positives in your life. Lalah Delia*

➤ *Stop hating yourself for everything you aren't. Start loving yourself for everything that you are. Unknown*

➤ *Self-love is asking yourself what you need—everyday—and then making sure you receive it. Unknown*

➤ *Of all the judgments we pass in life, none is more important than the judgment we pass on ourselves. Nathaniel Branden*

➤ *Song – "Broken Things" by Matthew West**

➤ *Song – "Hope in Front of Me" by Danny Gokey**

➤ *Song – "More Beautiful You" by Jonny Diaz**

➤ *Song – "You Are More" by Tenth Avenue North**

➤ *Song – "Greatest Love of All" by Whitney Houston**

Video available at https://bit.ly/2I38TXv

Reflect

1. Have you ever taken the time to try to describe yourself using only positive terms? Take the time now to list at least ten things. If you need help, ask others to describe you using only one positive word.

2. Have you ever experienced self-hatred? What have you done to overcome it?

3. Do you have a bully inside your head? What will it take to stand up for yourself and end the attacks?

4. Have you ever been through a time where you did whatever it took to survive only to experience shame and regret later?

5. Do you ever feel like no one understands what you're going through? No one understands why you made the choices you did? How does it make you feel to know God understands you?

6. Who are you? What makes you unique?

7. In the section Becoming a New Person, how did the phrases about the old you make you feel? Do you believe them? What would it take to believe them?

8. Are you ready to walk free from the chains of self-hatred?

9. Which Inspiration Suggestions did you choose to explore, and which stood out you'd like to remember?

10. What action steps do you need to take to implement what you've
    discovered in this chapter?

10

I Need to Learn How to Breathe

Coping Strategies

It has become very apparent the vast majority of what I've believed and thought for the past forty years was wrong. The way I've responded has been wrong. I've based all my actions and decisions on a skewed sense of reality. Though these things are painful to admit, along the way I've also discovered who I really am. Now it's time to start from scratch and rebuild my life the right way. But that means I need to start with the basics. How basic? Lord, teach me how to breathe!

The list below outlines the basics of everyday life. Day by day, minute by minute, and even, at times, second by second. I can honestly say, as ridiculous as some of these sound to me now, over a year after I was hospitalized, in the beginning I existed one second at a time, using these coping strategies repeatedly. At first, I had to be reminded to eat regularly and manage basic self-care.

Frequently, in a panic attack, I even needed to be reminded to breathe. This is not an exhaustive list on the topic of coping strategies. It's also not a professional list. It's my personal list. It's what got me through a time when I needed help to survive. I hope it will help you as well. I've included some action steps to help you personalize and use these strategies yourself.

Breathing

At times, even the simple act of breathing becomes a challenge. When I had difficulty processing a situation, my breathing would become rapid. As I stood shaking in fear, I could feel my heart beating as if it thought pounding hard enough and fast enough would allow it to escape from my chest. My entire focus at that moment was on finding a way to escape the situation.

Fight or flight? My mind didn't have the ability to face whatever was happening, so my body decided it needed a burst of adrenaline to either come to terms with my situation or run as fast as possible and find someplace safe to hide.

This fight-or-flight response happened multiple times a day at first, triggered by something as simple as someone I didn't know talking to me or being asked a question for which I didn't know the answer.

With help, I developed a series of steps to bring my breathing back under control. Someone would step directly in front of me and calmly say, "You're okay. Look at me. You're okay. Slow down your breathing. Breathe slowly with me, in through the nose and out through the mouth. Look at me. Breathe with me…"

They would continue to refocus me on three things: 1) I was okay; 2) I needed to keep my eyes focused on theirs; and 3) I needed to follow their slow breathing pattern. Sounds super simple because, honestly, it is. But it works! Or at least it did for me.

As my focus shifted from my problem to their face, to their words, to their breathing, my breathing slowed, and my heart rate followed suit. Eventually, I was able to use these steps as self-talk, which means I no longer need someone else to help me refocus. Now, I can talk to myself as a moment of panic comes over me and calm my own breathing.

> **ACTION STEP(S)**: Develop your own self-talk. Write down phrases that comfort you. Write down situations that might trigger the need for someone to talk you down from a heightened state of anxiety. Teach the above three steps, or your own self-talk script, to those close to you so they can help you when an occasion arises.

Thinking

"Don't copy the behaviors and customs of this world, but let God transform you into a new person by changing the way you think. Then you will learn to know God's will for you, which is good and pleasing and perfect." (Romans 12:2, NLT) This verse expresses the importance of what we think. The best way I've found to let God transform me into a new person is to start with a fresh mind each morning. Many people I know hit the snooze button in the morning to get that extra ten minutes of sleep. Others get out of bed and have a quiet time with God. I do a somewhat modified version of both.

When that sleep-shattering sound jolts me awake, I reach over and grope on the nightstand to find my phone. If I don't miss and knock it onto the floor, I unplug it from the charger and swipe it to silence the alarm. I already have a second alarm set for ten minutes later, and a third for ten minutes after that. I set the phone next to me on the bed and lay flat on my back in a relaxed position. Then I start to pray.

I spend the first few minutes of my prayer time focusing my mind on perspective, counting my many blessings, and thanking God for the abundant gifts he's given me. I continue by going through the prayer needs of others. I don't belabor each of them. God already knows their needs. I might simply say: be with Mark this week as he battles cancer or be with Heather as she searches for a job. If I have an area God has brought to my mind personally in my journey with him, I'll finish with that. I then go through a quick mental exercise, putting on the Armor of God. (Ephesians 6:10-17)

Now comes the hard part—getting out of bed and starting my day. I don't let the old negative thoughts or worries back in. I focus only on the positive, only on what is truth. As I focus on God's truth, his peace will fill me (Philippians 4:8). The minute I'm out the door, God's truth comes pouring into my heart through Christian radio. The songs I hear bring phrases and scripture to mind, which I then meditate on throughout the day.

Each night, I follow a similar routine of asking for grace for the many ways I've failed that day to keep my life aligned with God's will. You're shocked I'm sure to hear me say "many ways." Do you know how many times I get frustrated or short with other people each day? Or how many times I have jealous or prideful thoughts? By rewinding the tape of my day and confessing those shortcomings, I'm able to relax and feel renewed as I prepare to sleep and recharge.

When I started following this routine in the morning and evening, I started recognizing God's peace in my life. The struggles I faced seemed easier because I felt mentally prepared for battle. My faults throughout the day could be mentally processed and purged each night, so they didn't stick around and build up over time into a mountain of shortcomings that couldn't be overcome. My therapist has reminded me often, "Depression is living in the past, and anxiety is living in the future. Live where your feet are planted—in today, in the moment in front of you." By following this routine, I was able to do just that. I learned to live one day at a time.

ACTION STEP(S): Renew your mind daily. Develop a routine for starting and ending your day. In the morning, include time to count your blessings, focus your mind on the fresh start each day brings, and prepare spiritually for the battles ahead during the upcoming day by putting on the Armor of God. Memorize the protections of the Armor of God. Research what they mean if you're unsure. (e.g., breastplate of righteousness)

"Therefore, take up the full armor of God, so that you will be able to resist in the evil day, and having done everything, to stand firm. Stand firm therefore, *(1)* having girded your loins with truth, and having *(2)* put on the breastplate of righteousness, and having *(3)* shod your feet with the preparation of the gospel of peace; in addition to all, *(4)* taking up the shield of faith with which you will be able to extinguish all the flaming arrows of the evil one; and *(5)* take the helmet of salvation, and the *(6)* sword of the spirit, which is the word of God." Ephesians 6:10-17

In the evening, include time for reviewing your day for areas where you fell short of God's mark. Confess those actions, but more importantly, accept God's forgiveness. Before you will be able to rest and sleep, you must hear the words of Jesus to the adulteress woman, "Woman, where are they? Has no one condemned you?" "No one, sir," she said. "Then neither do I condemn you," Jesus declared. "Go now and leave your life of sin." (John 8:10-11)

Basic Self-Care

Basic daily habits like eating, drinking, and personal hygiene can easily be forgotten when you're depressed. In the hospital, we all went together to meals. I remember not wanting anything, but knew I had to eat it or they would come sit with me until I did. Every morning, we had to manage showers, dressing, and brushing our teeth. I know it doesn't seem like you should have to be reminded, but I did. When I first came home, my husband had to manage my medications and monitor my eating and sleeping habits. We'd go out to walk around the block to make sure I got some exercise.

All of these are very simple routine things the average person does on a daily basis without a thought. However, depression sufferers need a plan and an accountability partner until they can develop the ability to manage these tasks independently. It may require you to create a chart or reminder system. Set an alarm clock, if necessary, to make sure you get up and take care of yourself first thing in the morning. I promise—convincing yourself to get out of the bed is the hardest part. After you are up and moving, you just follow the same steps every day until it becomes habit.

> **ACTION STEP(S):** Develop a basic daily routine. Take a shower, brush your teeth, and brush your hair every morning. Include mealtimes and exercise. Find an accountability partner who will check up on you and monitor things for you until you're able to do it on your own. People want to help. Let them.

Emotional Care

I had a very difficult time keeping my emotions under control. I over-empathized with every pain of every person I saw in real life, on a TV show, or in a movie. Once the tears started, I was unable to stop them. I mean literally couldn't stop them until I was too physically exhausted to keep crying.

I would leave a situation halfway through if something triggered my emotions. We would turn off the TV or leave the theater if things overwhelmed me, and even then, I would continue to cry, unable to let it go.

Since the drama and family genres were off the table, we tried switching to action/adventure. Nope. Not good either. Every loud sound or sudden action would cause me to jump or tremble or start breathing heavily. I finally figured out a plan. Stick with comedy. Even if it didn't make me feel better, it at least didn't make me feel worse. I resigned myself to the fact that, at least for a time, I had to avoid negative, intense, or emotional situations. This included negative input from books, music, and movies.

> **ACTION STEP(S):** Surround yourself with positive people and

positive activities. Avoid stressful, emotional, and negative situations and people. If necessary, make a list. On a sheet of paper, draw a line across the top and then one down the middle to create a T-chart. Put the people and things that make you feel better on the left and those that bring you down on the right. Make time for the people and things on the left. You may need to, temporarily at least, step away from the people and things on the right.

Find a Christian radio station. If you are anything like me, spending hours every week in the car, the radio needs to have one station locked in. I challenge you to listen to a Christian radio station for thirty days and see if it doesn't make a positive difference in your thoughts and emotions. Don't just listen to the music; hear the words. Focus on a phrase throughout the day. Go online and find the lyrics to the songs. Learn them. Sing them. Absorb them into your heart and mind. Go to the artist's website and learn more about what scripture inspired them. Let God's words of truth invade your every thought whether through scripture or through music.

Spiritual Care

Get to know the God of the universe on a personal level. My depression led me to a crisis of faith. Learning to trust the God who held my life, my every breath, in his hand was critical for me. To overcome feelings of self-hate and unworthiness, I decided to see if what people had said about God loving the great men and women in the Bible, even when they screwed up, was true. I knew all the stories, but I did not know the whole story of some of these great men and woman.

I decided to read the Bible a little differently this time. I followed a chronological Bible reading plan. And I took notes. Lots of notes. Each person got a new page. I wrote down all the good, bad, and ugly in their lives. More importantly, I wrote down how God responded.

What I discovered was simple. It can be summed up in three short words. They were human. They had good days and bad, just like me. They had blessings and struggles, just like me. There were days I can honestly say the Bible was a real page-turner. Chronologically, it read like a novel. I literally couldn't put it down. The people came to life. I could truly relate to them. Many even had moments where they faced their own crisis of faith.

What I learned was this—God provided for them, continued to love them, and still used them to do great things. I learned I wasn't alone. I also learned God could be trusted. His character never changes. If he provided yesterday, he will provide today, and I can count on him to provide tomorrow.

Spending time each day in Bible study helped me focus my thoughts on the size of my God, rather than the size of my circumstances. That perspective is critical. Each day is a brand-new opportunity to acknowledge God and all his work on my behalf in the past, at present, and for the future. Joy and peace come from continued trust in God. (Romans 15:13)

When I trust him, and then see him come through day after day in my life and the lives of those around me, it gives me the peace and joy that come from knowing God has everything under control. He'll be there when I need him. It's only as I'm able to feel that peace and joy grow stronger within me that I'm able to overcome depression and start living the abundant life that God intended.

ACTION STEP(S): Schedule time each day, preferably early in the day, for prayer and study of God's Word. Find a Bible study you like and commit to it. Or make a decision to start reading through the Bible. I recommend a chronological study. For me, it seemed more like a typical off-the-shelf book you might read where things go in order and context makes it easier to understand things. Get to know the God of the universe who loves you and has a plan for your life.

Make a list of all the people in the Bible whose names you may already know, such as Abraham, Isaac, Jacob and so on. Next, write down all the times they failed in their lives. Finally, write the many blessings God bestowed on them in spite of their mistakes and poor choices. Refer back to this list when you feel you are not worthy of God's forgiveness and blessing. I promise you will soon realize your mistakes and poor choices fit right in with all the people in the Bible through whom God did extraordinary things.

Journaling

When I got settled in my room at the hospital, they brought me a standard black-and-white composition notebook. It was for me to write my thoughts in, they explained. As I sat and stared at the blank pages, I wondered not only about what to write, but how I could possibly ever fill all those pages. It started out to be a typical "Dear Diary..." where I described every detail of my day from what I ate to what I did. Snooze!

But it evolved. I started writing what I was thinking about and what questions I had. I described emotions and wondered about what triggered them. I started to analyze rather than report my life. I took the time to process things that were happening and how I felt about them. These writings allowed me to develop a plan of action to avoid similar problems in the future. It also allowed me to look back and see how much I'd already overcome.

ACTION STEP(S): End each day processing the good, the bad, and the ugly parts of your day. Find the blessings hidden within all of it. Write out your challenges and brainstorm a plan for overcoming them. Write out your successes and celebrate them.

Identify Your Triggers

Don't let people push your buttons. Think to yourself:

- Why did they do that? Maybe something is going on with them, and it isn't about you at all.

- Why did what they do or say upset me?

- How did I handle it? How could I handle it differently?

- How could I keep from letting them push my buttons in the future if this situation comes up again?

- What caused me to react the way I did?

The answer to that last question is simple. It's called an automatic thought. Automatic thoughts are any "thoughts that automatically come to mind when a particular situation occurs."[1] It's like when the doctor taps on your knee and your lower leg jumps. It's an automatic response to a specific trigger.

But, what's the trigger that is causing the negative thoughts? That's where journaling helps. Ask yourself:

- What happened right before my emotional response?

- Is what's happening rational? Is it true?

- How can I look at it differently or more positively?

Once you determine what's triggering your reaction, you can work to create a new response. Identifying triggers and changing behavior is the primary focus of Cognitive Behavioral Therapy. A good psychologist, behavioral therapist, or Licensed Mental Health Counselor can help with this process.

I can certainly attest to the fact that a good Christian therapist is truly worth the time and effort it takes to find them. I'll admit, there are days I leave a session mad because she won't just tell me how to fix whatever's wrong. But when she forces me to figure out how to fix things on my own, the feeling is very empowering.

There are days I leave a session sad because she speaks truth I'm not ready to hear and don't want to admit. But I always discover she's right when I put the effort into processing her words and accept their truth. Overall, I've grown so much over the last year solely through the grace of God and the work my therapist has made me do. I realize what a true blessing she has been. (Thank you, Kelly!)

ACTION STEP(S): Make a Trigger List. As you recognize new triggers, add them to your Trigger List and develop a plan for how to deal with them.

Find a local psychologist, behavioral therapist, or Licensed Mental Health Counselor and make an appointment. Follow up regularly for as long as it takes. After a few sessions, if you do not feel a connection with them, consider finding someone else. Pray God will lead you to the right therapist. Once there, do the work. Process your thoughts, feelings, and actions for as long as it takes to make changes.

Awareness

Be aware of your actions and reactions. While this is very similar to identifying your triggers, it's not exactly the same. As I work daily to renew my mind, I pray for God to guide me to see my behavior through his eyes in a specific area of my life. For instance, remember how I mentioned all the things my husband used to do that annoyed me, and then when I realized his unconditional love for me, they didn't seem so annoying? Well, unfortunately he does still annoy me from time to time; after all, he's not perfect. So one day I prayed God would give me the strength to offer grace rather than engage in the typical negative dialog that previously would've caused me to pull away.

Later that morning, I was reminded of a phrase I'd heard several times before about working to win the relationship rather than the argument. I remembered that phrase all day long. I thought about ways I could change my actions/reactions to avoid bitter, resentful feelings, which is how I'd always dealt with it in the past. Once again, I prayed God would give me the strength to offer grace.

That evening, my husband was particularly annoying. I remember saying to God in my frustration, "I didn't ask you to give me opportunities to learn how to offer grace. I asked you to give me the strength to offer it."

It was almost as if I heard angels singing in the background as I very clearly heard God speak to my heart, "You have to learn how to offer grace before I can strengthen your ability to offer it."

My shoulders sank, and I breathed out a long, hard half-laugh, half-sigh at those words. I realized I'd been asking God to give me something I was apparently unwilling to put in the effort to learn on my own.

What does this have to do with awareness, you ask? When I prayed for God's help dealing with my husband, he chose instead to help me be more aware of my own behavior and my role in changing it and, subsequently, the situation. Fortunately, that awareness has continued. Have I started offering grace constantly? No. Have I had more opportunities to learn grace? Absolutely.

I'm frequently reminded of what Jesus told his disciples about being judgmental. "Why do you look at the speck of sawdust in your brother's eye and pay no attention to the plank in your own eye?" (Matthew 7:3) Ouch!

I can already hear what's coming next, and it certainly applies to me in this situation. Jesus says in verse 5, "You hypocrite." Double ouch! By focusing my attention on my behavior, rather than my husband's, I've been allowed to see the plank in my own eye. My awareness has been placed squarely on the one and only thing I can change. Me.

ACTION STEP(S): Pray daily God will bring awareness of what in your life isn't in line with his will. Then open your eyes, your mind, and your heart to his answer.

As you become aware of areas where you might need some work, don't stop there. Knowing there's an area that doesn't align with God's will isn't enough. This brings us back to journaling. Write down things God's brought to your mind.

Then pray daily God will give you opportunities to learn how to become more like him in that area. Most importantly, follow through. Write down ways your actions and reactions might be different and practice them over and over until they become part of you.

Memorize Philippians 4:6-9.

Do not be anxious about anything, but in every situation, by prayer and petition, with thanksgiving, present your requests to God. And the peace of God, which transcends all understanding, will guard your hearts and your minds in Christ Jesus. Finally, brothers and sisters, whatever is true, whatever is noble, whatever is right, whatever is pure, whatever is lovely, whatever is admirable—if anything is excellent or praiseworthy—think about such things. Whatever you have learned or received or heard from me, or seen in me—put it into practice. And the God of peace will be with you.

Healthy Detachment

The blessings and hardships of others don't affect me. When a friend is suffering a medical crisis, I can empathize with their pain and pray for relief. When someone makes a poor choice, which is followed by consequences, I can empathize with their situation and pray for grace.

However, in either situation, what I can't do is fix it. That's where my issue with codependency comes in. I'm not God. I have absolutely no control over their situations. It's not my problem to fix. I didn't cause it, and I can't save them from whatever's coming next. In reality, it doesn't affect my life at all; yet, I still spend sleepless nights trying to figure out how to help.

In the same way, when someone receives good news financially, or in their career, all I can do is be happy for them. What someone else has that I don't have is irrelevant. Remember that tenth commandment, Thou shalt not covet? (Exodus 20:17)

I'll admit that it's particularly hard not to covet when others take advantage of the system and are handed everything they've ever wanted when I've struggled for everything I have. When that happens, I refer back to Philippians 4:19, where I'm reminded God will supply all my needs. I've looked hard at that one. Nowhere in there does it talk about wants.

I have all I need. I have food, water, and shelter. I have the ability to breathe and the mental capacity to reason. And, most importantly, I have the love of the God of the universe. Sometimes I just have to remind myself of this fact—there's nothing anyone else has that I want more than I want Jesus. No amount of money or things could ever replace Jesus in my life. I'm learning to acknowledge God for what I have and ask how I can use it for his glory.

ACTION STEP(S): Keep a prayer journal. It can be as simple or elaborate as you desire. Keep track of every person and situation for which you pray. Use it when you pray. Yes, it's okay to open your eyes and look at it as you pray. Remember to write answers to prayers as well.

Create a Blessings Jar. Every time a blessing comes to your mind, write it on a small scrap of paper, or a notecard, and place it in the jar. These reminders will help you focus on all the many things God has done for you. When you are feeling down about something, these blessing slips will provide that extra little reminder you need to keep your eyes focused on your eternal God and not your temporary situation.

When we get back to the basics and realize it all starts with breathing, we realize we never learned how to breathe—we just did it. At the moment we were born, we began breathing. That's the sign of life for which every parent waits, that first cry from their newborn baby. The sound that demonstrates the baby is taking air in and forcing it back out. Breathing. If God gave us the ability to do that, he'll also give us the ability to do everything else that comes up. Quit trying to do things on your own and just focus on him.

Inspiration Suggestions

> *Your breathing is your greatest friend. Return to it in all your troubles and you will find comfort and guidance. Unknown*

142

➢ *Taking care of your mind, body, and spirit—also known as self-care—is one of the most important things you can do for your long-term health. Anita Sun*

➢ *I'm still coping with my trauma, but coping by trying to find different ways to heal it rather than hide it. Clemantine Wamariya*

➢ *Something wonderful begins to happen with the simple realization that life, like an automobile, is driven from the inside out, not the other way around. Richard Carlson*

➢ *Don't copy the behavior and customs of this world, but let God transform you into a new person by changing the way you think. Then you will learn to know God's will for you, which is good and pleasing and perfect. Romans 12:2*

➢ *Relying on God has to start all over every day, as if nothing has yet been done. C.S. Lewis*

➢ *Song – "Cast My Cares" by Finding Favour**

➢ *Song – "Warrior" by Hannah Kerr**

*Video available at https://bit.ly/2I38TXv

Reflect

1. Have you ever experienced a panic attack and needed help with something as simple as breathing?

2. Do you have a routine for renewing your mind every morning and evening? If not, what would you include in it?

3. Do you take good care of yourself? Do you track your self-care

habits to make sure you're doing the things that will keep you healthy and keep your mind off of your depression?

4. How well do you manage your emotions? Is there an activity or person you need to step away from for a time?

5. How often do you spend time getting to know the God of the entire universe? How can you get to know him better?

6. What can you do differently to increase your trust in God by learning more about him?

7. Have you ever taken the time to identify what triggers your emotions? What do you feel would be the best way to do that?

8. Do you use a journal? How can you spend more time reflecting rather than reporting? What can you do differently to plan for change when your reflection shows a need for it?

9. Do you ever feel like no one understands what you're going through? No one understands why you made the choices you did? How does it make you feel to know God understands you?

10. Which Inspiration Suggestions did you choose to explore, and which stood out you'd like to remember?

11. What action steps do you need to take to implement what you've discovered in this chapter?

11

I Need to Live in the Moment

Surviving

I passed the class! I have all the knowledge and skills to beat depression. I even have a certificate to prove it. Now what?

Once I was back in the real world, I very quickly discovered knowledge and skills didn't count for anything if I couldn't use them in a moment of crisis. Which for me, at that point, was pretty much every moment that came by. Knowing and doing are two distinctly different things.

Just because I knew what to do didn't mean I could actually do it. In real time. The first time. I reacted just like a baby learning to walk. Babies know what to do; they've seen everyone around them do it their entire lives. Putting it into practice on command is a little more elusive. It seems like every time they try, they fall. But over time they get steadier, stronger, and farther along in the process. Until finally, they walk.

Unfortunately, I didn't have the luxury of unlimited time and space to do nothing but practice my new skill. The world wasn't going to slow to my pace while I practiced surviving on my own. But in order to win the war against depression, I had to fight one step, one fall, one minute at a time.

Using Your Coping Skills

There are a million and one coping strategies out there. I outlined several of the ones that worked for me in the previous chapter.

Just because I knew what to do didn't mean I could actually do it. In real time. The first time.

These strategies took time and practice to master. Trying to get up and walk again after being struck down by depression is an overwhelming process. There are so many things to remember and do to keep from falling again. Remembering everything at the same time is virtually impossible. For me, the number one coping skill I had to remember, and master, was breathing.

I quickly discovered how much anxiety I felt when I didn't know how to respond to something. Not big things, really. Little things, like being around people. It didn't matter who at that point. Seeing or even hearing anyone but my husband was paralyzing.

Someone would call to check on me or stop by to see if I was ok. My throat would tighten up, locking each fresh breath of air out of my lungs, while my heart began to pound against my chest. My hands refused to be still, and I felt frozen in place, even though my mind kept screaming at me to run. I learned if I didn't handle that anxiety quickly, at the first pound of my heart or gasp for breath, it would turn in to a full-blown panic attack.

While panic attacks themselves are not fatal, I know failing to have a heartbeat or take a breath are. That became my priority. I didn't know how to force my heart to stop pounding, but I'd learned how to slow down my breathing, which made it easier to take air into my lungs.

It's this exact principle that guides triage centers. Deal with the lifesaving measures first and move on from there. You can come back to the lesser issues later. It's extremely difficult to think clearly when your brain isn't receiving the proper amount of oxygen, or at least that's what we've told kids at test time for all the years I've been in education.

Learning to Breathe

So that's where I started—learning to breathe in the midst of panic. My first experience actually happened before I got out of the hospital. I'd been released from inpatient care and was participating in the outpatient partial hospitalization program.

One day, a young man said something that went completely against everything I knew to be true about God. I wanted to scream and shout at him that he was wrong. I knew I had to speak up but wasn't sure I could. That's when I felt it coming on. The panic rose up in me until I couldn't contain it.

I managed to speak the truth in spurts as I willed myself to breathe in as deeply as I could. As my hands began to shake, my voice did as well. The tears began to fall, and my heart pounded so intensely that I thought it would explode along with my anger. Then, I ran.

I knocked over chairs and pushed people who were in my way until I was able to exit the room into the hall. I looked left—dead end. I looked right—doorway to the front lobby of the hospital where an employee was walking towards me. Straight across was a short hallway with an office on either side. I ran into the hallway, put my back to the wall, covered my eyes, and slid down the wall in a heap of tears and sobs.

That's where the therapist found me. It was probably only seconds later, but it certainly seemed much longer. I vaguely remember hearing her through the explosion of my rapidly beating heart. I remember hearing her completely calm voice amidst my hysteria, almost whispering, "Look at me."

When I finally worked up enough courage to uncover my eyes to look at her, she whispered, "You're okay." I could still feel my body shaking and felt like I could hear my heart exploding within me. My sobs were like crashing waves, one on top of the other, thundering so loudly they almost drowned out her still, calm voice.

I kept trying to avert my eyes from hers, feeling overwhelmed and embarrassed by the judgment she must feel about the scene I was causing. Each time I tried, her hushed "Look at me" drew me back. No judgment in those eyes. Again, she said, "You're okay."

As she saw I could no longer look away, she said, "Slow down your breathing. Breathe with me, in through the nose and out through the mouth." She then inhaled deeply through her nose and exhaled slowly and loudly through her mouth as if forcing every ounce of oxygen in her lungs to leave her body.

She continued to breathe slowly saying, "Breathe with me. Come on, you can do it." My first attempts failed as the air rushed in and out of my mouth at a record-setting pace. She kept coaching and willing me with every fiber of her being to slow down.

I'm not sure when it happened, but it did. My breathing became slow and steady just like hers. We sat there in that hallway just breathing for who knows how long before she finally touched me. She softly put her hand on my shoulder and said, "See! I told you you were okay." And she smiled. Those nonjudgmental, compassionate eyes smiled. I had no choice but to do the same.

That was my first experience using a coping skill in real time. It worked. So well, in fact, it was the first thing I told my husband when I got in the car that afternoon. I had hope and couldn't wait to share it. I told him he had one job in life, and then I explained the simple procedure the therapist had followed to bring me back from the brink of hysteria to reality.

I wasn't sure what the next moment would bring, but I did know that, at least for that moment, I was alive, I was breathing, and I was okay.

Sound ridiculous? Sound too simple? It *is* simple, but that's where I needed to start. That's how I survived that one moment. I wasn't sure what the next moment would bring, but I did know that, at least for that moment, I was alive, I was breathing, and I was okay.

That strategy wasn't the only one that helped me as I encountered plenty of new moments in my journey towards recovery. If it was the only one, Chapter 9 wouldn't exist. No two moments in my day were the same. Each situation I found myself in required new skills to cope with them. A few weeks later I found myself in another dilemma.

Breathing in Real Time

It was supposed to be a relaxing night. We invited two couples, our dearest friends, to come over for dinner and some games. Remember I mentioned earlier how little things like being around other people were difficult for me? I was very anxious about how I would do but knew I needed to stretch myself. After all, they loved me dearly and wanted nothing more than to love on me and help me get better. How could anything go wrong?

My husband took care of everything in preparation for their arrival. He cleaned the house and prepared dinner. All I had to do was show up and not lose it. Well, at least I mastered half of that.

It was awkward at first. No one really knew what to do or say, but we got into a comfortable rhythm of conversation. After dinner, I was feeling more relaxed. We started to play games. My friends brought a game where a person gives you clues, and you have to guess the word they're describing. It came complete with a little timer you passed around as you took your turn.

As the timer gets handed from one person to the next, the beeps get faster and faster until it explodes with a loud buzzer noise. In hindsight, probably not the wisest game choice for someone in my fragile emotional state.

I don't even have to describe what happened because I'm sure you can guess. As the timer sped up, so did my breathing. My heart rate followed suit until my entire body was in a state of high anxiety. I jumped up from the table and ran into my room, slamming the door behind me.

I didn't want my husband to leave our company, drawing even more attention to my inability to survive even this simple, enjoyable evening with friends. However, he has a mind of his own. As he quietly entered the room with compassion and concern on his face, I waved him off, unable yet to speak through my gasping breath. He stood indecisive for a moment and then walked back out quietly, closing the door and leaving me to myself.

I knew what I needed to do. I needed to calm myself. But could I do it on my own? Like a sleepy, crying child in the dark hours of the night, I needed to figure out how to self-soothe.

Learning to Self-Soothe

I rummaged through the folder of notes from the group therapy sessions until I found my exit strategy plan from my inpatient stay. I rapidly scanned down the list of strategies I could use until I found the one I sought. Soft music calms the soul.

I remembered one group session where we listened to soft instrumental music to calm ourselves. We closed our eyes and tried to make sense of the music. What picture did it bring to mind? How did it make us feel? The leader kept saying, "Focus on the music, nothing else. Breathe slowly, in and out." I sensed a common theme there.

I left my papers and found my phone, clicked on the music app, and located the station I had pre-programmed for meditation. It's what I affectionately call elevator music. I lay down on the bed in a comfortable position, closed my eyes and tried to focus on the music as I'd been taught. But my mind kept jumping back to the friends in the other room.

No!

Stop!

Focus on the music! What do you see? How does it make you feel?

This process repeated numerous times until I finally realized I was breathing a little more slowly. I was able to focus on the music and the calm melody blowing over me like a breeze over a field of spring flowers on a sunny day. How anxious can you be with that picture in your head? Again, simple? Yes, very simple. But it worked.

Both these strategies continued to get a workout as I lived moment by moment over the next few months. I'd learned how to bring my body back under control most of the time, but who wants to go through life controlling their reactions? I didn't want to react to situations. I wanted to learn how to be proactive.

Journaling was critical for me at this point. Each night, and sometimes several times during the day, I processed my activities and emotions by writing in my journal. Not only did I analyze what I was doing and why I might be doing it, it was also a way for me to lay it down before the Lord. I know when I give my burdens to the Lord, he won't let me slip or fall. (Psalm 55:22) Giving things to God—another coping skill I'm trying to learn.

You Win Some, You Lose Some

Sure, in the beginning, emotional situations came up that threw me off balance, and I fell into old habits. Before I had time to journal about it, or analyze why I couldn't handle it, the anxiety train had left the station, run me over, and gotten halfway to its destination while another train stood in its place ready to flatten me again.

Learning to survive moment by moment in real time comes in stages. It's a process.

At first, you may not even recognize your mistake. Others may need to bring it to your attention. Otherwise, you just sit and suffer the consequences.

At some point, you start recognizing your mistake, but not soon enough to take action to prevent it. You still suffer the consequences, but usually you can resolve things sooner with the knowledge and awareness of the problem.

Eventually, you start learning to recognize the signs and symptoms that a problem is on the horizon prior to it actually happening. Sometimes you realize in time, and sometimes you don't, but you make progress in the right direction.

> *You win some, you lose some. But, eventually, you win way more often than you lose.*

Finally, you come to a point where you no longer have to watch for signs and symptoms of an impending problem, you just know what to do, and you proactively prevent the problem from occurring.

You win some, you lose some. But eventually, you win way more often than you lose.

It was the same with my emotions. Sometimes I was able to use a coping strategy and manage the issue on my own. Other times, it was completely out of my control.

God Is in Control

It was pretty clear to everyone at this point in my recovery that I wasn't in control. I was still in stage one—I often didn't even recognize there was a problem until it was too late. For the first time in my life, I realized I didn't want to be in control, and I wasn't afraid of what might happen if I wasn't in control.

I knew for certain this situation was way beyond me or any skills I might possess. It was time to acknowledge I was fighting against evil rulers and authorities of the unseen world. It was time to put on every piece of God's armor in order to resist the enemy so that, after the battle, I would be standing firm. (Ephesians 6:12-13) It was time to acknowledge that by trusting God and using the armor he provided for me to protect myself, I could overcome any obstacle in my way as I sought to achieve victory over depression.

When I struggle with turning over control, I remember the words of God to Jeremiah as he faced the Babylonian attack against Jerusalem. He said, "I am the Lord, the God of all mankind. Is anything too hard for me?" (Jeremiah 32:27)

Jeremiah knew God was taking the Israelites into a time of captivity, but he also knew God was in control and trusted his plan. The question is always, can I do the same? Can I trust God's in control? Can I trust he's enough?

When I ask these questions silently in my mind, the words of Twila Paris'

"God Is in Control" come rushing out with every ounce of confidence I have within me. I can trust in God's plan. I can't allow my emotions to lead me astray or cause me to lose my focus on him. I can trust in God's promises because he never changes. It's no wonder the song won the Gospel Music Association's Song of the Year award. It's a fight song for those who're struggling.

One ~~Day~~ Minute at a Time

The struggle with depression is a daily battle to be won. It starts with mastering one minute at a time. Soon it will be thirty or sixty minutes at a time without having to think what to do. I know that sounds ridiculous, but for those living it, like me, what an accomplishment.

Then hours will become days and weeks until you finally realize you're headed towards your new victorious life. Unfortunately, as with any new skill, I fell. You'll fall, too.

There were moments when I asked myself, "How did I get back down here." There will be days when for every three steps you take forward you end up taking two steps back. But do the math! That's still one step in the right direction. You're still moving forward! You may lose a few battles along the way. Keep at it, and you WILL win the war.

Inspiration Suggestions

➢ *We gain strength and courage and confidence by each experience in which we really stop to look fear in the face . . . we must do that which we think we cannot. Eleanor Roosevelt*

➢ *You can't stop the waves, but you can learn to surf. Jon Kabot-Zinn*

➢ *Wake up knowing that whatever happens today, you can handle it. Unknown*

➢ *Be gentle with yourself. You're doing the best you can. Unknown*

➢ *I'm still coping with my trauma, but coping by trying to find different ways to heal it rather than hide it. Clemantine Wamariya*

➢ *Nothing can bring you peace but yourself. Ralph Waldo Emerson*

➢ *Today I will not stress over things I can't control. Unknown*

➢ *You're not going to master the rest of your life in one day. Just relax. Master the day. Then just keep doing that every day. Unknown*

➢ *I will breathe. I will think of solutions. I will not let worry control me. I will not let my stress level break me. I will simply breathe, and it will be okay because I don't quit. Shayne McClendon*

➢ *Song – "Breathe" by Jonny Diaz**

➢ *Song – "Lord, I Need You" by Matt Maher**

➢ *Song – "Overcomer" by Mandisa**

➢ *Song – "Stronger" by Mandisa**

*Video available at https://bit.ly/2I38TXv

Reflect

1. What's the biggest struggle you face for which you need to find a coping strategy to help you survive?

2. What coping strategies have you used? Have they helped?

3. Have you ever practiced controlling your breathing under stress? How did it make you feel? Can you do it on command?

4. Have you discussed with your friends and family how they can help

155

in a time of crisis? Have you taught them what works for you? Have you ever practiced calming yourself by listening to soft music and meditating on what it makes you see in your mind and how it makes you feel? How did it make you feel? Can you do it on command?

5. Have you ever tried journaling as a way to identify your emotional triggers, process your feelings, and track your progress? What did you like and dislike about the process? What could you do to make it a better tool for you in the future?

6. Do you regularly practice giving your worries and cares over to God in prayer? And leaving them there with him to handle? How do you think that practice might help you?

7. In which stage of the change process do you find yourself: oblivious there even is a problem, recognizing it after the fact, or recognizing it in time to be proactive?

8. What steps can you take to move yourself forward in this process of change from reactive to proactive?

9. Are you familiar with the Armor of God? If not, what can you do to learn how to use it to overcome daily struggles?

10. Do you truly believe nothing is too difficult for God? What would it take to believe that? What steps can you take to become more

familiar with God's power over evil and how he can help you with your struggles?

11. Are you able to fully trust God is in control of everything in your life? What would it take for you to be able to trust him in all circumstances?

12. Which Inspiration Suggestions did you choose to explore, and which stood out you'd like to remember?

13. What action steps do you need to take to implement what you've discovered in this chapter?

12

I Need a New Direction

Plan B

Whenever my mother asked what was going on, I'd always respond, "Well, the plan is…" She'd chuckle and say, "I can count on the fact you always have a plan." Little did she realize I was simply following in her footsteps.

My mom has always been a list maker. Everything is always planned out in advance and well organized. For instance, she had a list of camping supplies broken down by which camping box they went in. She later had a similar list for the motor home, which I'm sure was probably broken down by the compartment in which things would be stored. She had a list for trips broken down by what clothing, jewelry, and toiletries to bring. And the biggest list of all is her inheritance list. This list contains practically everything in her home of value and states the origin, history, estimated value, and who it will go to upon her death. Her lists take the concept of planning ahead to a whole new level.

Don't even get me started on the calendar. If it wasn't on the calendar, it didn't happen. Our life seemed ruled by the Girl Scout calendar that always hung on the wall in the kitchen.

When my husband and I first married, it was obvious opposites do, in fact, attract. Like my mother, I had every moment of every day for the next six months planned out and budgeted, while my husband didn't know what he was going to do for dinner.

I brought my mom's calendar habit into my family by having a Sunday night family meeting. If it didn't get talked about at that meeting and put on the calendar, it didn't happen. Don't tell me you need a tri-fold board for your science fair project on Wednesday night when it's due on Thursday. Sorry! Plan ahead!

Unfortunately, plans don't do any good if you're planning for the wrong thing.

My Ladder Was Against the Wrong Wall

Many experts in the field of organization and time management stress the importance of this obsession with planning and recordkeeping. Steven R. Covey's book *Seven Habits of Highly Effective People* has been a staple on my bookshelf for decades. I've read it multiple times and refer to it often for reminders. In Habit Two, "Begin with the End in Mind," Covey states, "If your ladder is not leaning against the right wall, every step you take gets you to the wrong place faster."

> *If you don't consciously think about, plan, and live out the life you desire, you have, by default, given that very precious power to those around you and to the day-to-day experiences you have along the way.*

His premise is, if you don't consciously think about, plan, and live out the life you desire, you have, by default, given that very precious power to those around you and to the day-to-day experiences you have along the way.

As I said earlier, I've always had a plan. I consciously work hard to find a way to make that plan work out. However, I also truly believe God has a better plan for my life than I ever could. He has every day of my life mapped out with the end in mind, eternity with him. My responsibility for being involved in that plan is to stay focused on the plan, consciously and actively living it out one minute at a time. But how does that work when I have my own plans?

Have you ever taken a plane trip to see a loved one? My son lives in Seattle, and I live in Florida, so a plane trip is really my only way to see him. If I get on a plane here in Orlando with plans to see my son in Seattle, I full

160

well expect, and rightfully so, to get off the plane in Seattle. If the pilot shares my interest in going to Seattle, and takes off with that plan in mind, we all feel like things should go as expected. Right?

Well, once in the sky, other forces act on that plane to divert it from its intended course. There are winds, storms, birds, and other planes, which all impact which path we might take. Obviously, the invention of automatic pilot has made these obstacles much less of an issue. However, if the pilot doesn't stay focused on his instruments, heed the warnings they might give, then consciously and actively make constant course corrections, we may end up in Los Angeles instead of Seattle. While Los Angeles is beautiful, it's not where I wanted to find myself at the end of this trip.

The same is true of my life. God has had a plan for my life from long before I was even born. As David declared in Psalm 139:16, "You saw me before I was born. Every day of my life was recorded in your book. Every moment was laid out before a single day had passed."

Just like my expectation is for the pilot to stick to the plan of getting me to Seattle, God's expectation is for me to consciously stick to his plan. However, I failed. The experiences I had along the way in my life distracted me and sent me off course. Forget Los Angeles, I missed the mark by so much I ended up in Mexico.

While Mexico, and Los Angeles, are great places to be, they aren't where I wanted to be. I wanted to be spending time with my son. Because I wasn't focused on checking my status as I went through life to see if I was on track, because I wasn't making constant course corrections, I didn't reach my final destination. I reached somewhere I didn't really want to be. I climbed the ladder to success, or at least what I thought was success, only to find it didn't lead me to where I wanted to go.

The ladder of success the world told me I needed to climb was definitely not leaning against the right wall, or even the right building. How do I know that? I got to the top, stepped out onto the roof, and looked around. I very quickly discovered that where I was standing looked nothing like where I wanted to be. The place where I knew I belonged.

> *I climbed the ladder to success, or at least what I thought was success, only to find it didn't lead me to where I wanted to go.*

Unfortunately, it wasn't until I climbed that ladder, got to the top, looked around, and discovered I was way off target that I realized much of my life had passed me by. That begs the question, "Why did God take so long to step in and fulfill his plans for my life?"

God's Plan Finally Fulfilled for Abraham

In the book of Genesis, we are introduced to Abraham. He was a man filled with faith in God and in his promises. At God's calling, and at the age of seventy-five, Abraham left his homeland for places God promised to show him. Even though he and his wife, Sarah, had no children, God promised, "I will give this land to your descendants." (Genesis 12:7)

Keep in mind, people lived to a much older age than we do and had children at a much older age as well. Having a child at seventy-five wasn't completely impossible, which probably helped Abraham believe God's promise without questioning God's timing.

Years later, after Abraham and Lot, his nephew, had parted ways, God again told Abraham, "I am giving all this land, as far as you can see, to you and your descendants as a permanent possession." (Geneses 13:15) There's that descendants word again.

At this point, still childless, Abraham was beginning to doubt God would come through on his promise. He asked, "What good are all your blessings when I don't even have a son?"

He went on to tell God he would need to have an heir through his servant, since Sarah was barren, to which God replied, "You will have a son of your own who will be your heir." Though it really seemed impossible at this point, Abraham believed God's promise and Genesis 15:2-5 tells us his faith was counted as righteousness. Abraham has believed God for close to a decade by now, without question, so why is his belief just now counted as righteous?

I believe God knew Abraham was really starting to doubt the promise would ever be fulfilled. While childbirth at seventy-five may have been possible, as the years passed, it was less and less probable. However, despite his doubt, he still chose to believe God's promise. That's what faith means—believing in spite of our doubt.

Sarah also became discouraged and doubted the promise would ever be fulfilled, so she devised a plan to help provide an heir. She offers up her maidservant, who becomes pregnant and delivers Abraham, at the age of eighty-six, a son named Ishmael.

However, God didn't need Sarah's help to give Abraham a son. This was their plan, not God's plan. They tried to force God's plan to happen rather than waiting on God's timing, which is why Ishmael's life would be a constant source of conflict in Abraham's life.

God didn't punish Abraham or Sarah for getting off track or for thinking their plan was better than his. He did, however, allow them to suffer the natural consequences of having a child by a woman who is not your wife.

When Abraham was ninety-nine years old, God appeared to him again and promised, if Abraham would serve him faithfully and live a blameless life, he would give him countless descendants to whom the land of Canaan would belong forever.

That's what is called a covenant, which in this case was an agreement between God and the ancient Israelites, in which God promised to protect them if they kept his law and were faithful to him.

That covenant outlined how God would bless Abraham, and what he and his descendants needed to do to receive that blessing. God said, "Your responsibility is to obey the terms of the covenant. You and all your descendants have this continual responsibility." (Genesis 17:9) Verse 10 goes on to outline some very specific terms for this specific covenant.

Why do I bring up the responsibility of obeying the terms of the agreement, which in this case was to have all males circumcised, when I'm talking about God's promises for me and his plan for my life? This covenant represented a very specific promise to a very specific person. Many would say I can't even apply it to my life.

> *We have a responsibility to obey in order to receive his blessings.*

However, as I've said before—and I stand by it still—God never changes. His character is always the same and he can be trusted to stay the same. His expectations are the same for all of us. It's simple; we have a responsibility to obey in order to receive his blessings.

In terms of God's plan for my life, that responsibility to obey means I need to consciously and actively live in a way that fulfills his plan for my life, which is to spend eternity with him. Covenants are two-way agreements. When I'm not fulfilling my end of the agreement, I can't expect God to fulfill his. Each has a responsibility.

God is very clear about this. "Any male who fails to be circumcised will be cut off from the covenant family for breaking the covenant." (Genesis 17:14) In essence, God was saying he absolutely wants to bless us. In exchange, he expects us to invest some effort in that blessing by doing what we are asked. By obeying.

Abraham invested some effort into receiving God's blessing. He did what God asked and was circumcised himself along with all the members of his household. God, true to his word, fulfilled his promise to Abraham. Sarah went on to give birth to Isaac, who did indeed go on to bring Abraham countless descendants. However, Abraham had to wait twenty-five years for the fulfillment of God's promise.

Those years were at times filled with doubt and disobedience. They were also filled with unpleasant consequences for not following God's plan. I imagine Abraham might have benefitted from the words penned much later in Proverbs 3:5-6, "Trust in the Lord with all your heart; do not depend on your own understanding. Seek his will in all you do, and he will show you which path to take."

God's Plan Finally Fulfilled for Joshua

Joshua, another man of God, was leading the Israelites after their forty years of wandering in the desert was complete. Once again, God called for the Israelites to be circumcised to recommit them to God's promises to bless them and bring them into the land of Canaan. Once they'd made this recommitment to obey God, he blessed them with a sound victory over Jericho without a single battle.

Feeling confident and courageous with their newfound power to defeat the enemy, they made a fatal mistake. They were filled with pride and confidence in their own ability to defeat their enemies. Some would even say they became cocky, thinking they only had to show up and God would do the rest. As they continued their journey to conquer the land of Canaan with their puffed-up egos, they headed into a second city, Ai, with too few men and were soundly defeated, running away in fear.

Joshua and his men, who thought they understood God's plan, fell to their faces on the ground, crying out to him in doubt saying, "Why did you bring us across the Jordan River if you are going to let the Amorites kill us?" In other words, we thought you wanted us to take this land for you; why didn't you work your magic again?

God responded, "Get up! Why are you lying on your face? Israel has sinned and broken my covenant." (Joshua 7:6-11)

There's that word again. Covenant. The two-way agreement.

God reprimanded them, telling them they hadn't done what was expected of them. Therefore, God wouldn't bless them. God goes on to say, "You will never defeat your enemies until you remove these things from among you." (Joshua 7:13)

Again, a specific promise and a specific expectation, but the underlying principle is the same. God expects us to obey him.

Just as Abraham before him did, Joshua corrected the sin among the people. He once again made things right with God. God, in turn, goes on to say, "Do not be afraid or discouraged. Take all your fighting men and attack Ai, for I have given you the king of Ai, his people, his town, and his land." (Joshua 8:1)

God kept his promise and soundly defeated the city and people of Ai. Joshua originally chose to follow his own plan at Ai, thinking he knew what was best. As a result, he was soundly defeated. He comes back at God with doubt and disappointment, wondering what happened, since he thought defeating the city was what God wanted. And it was. However, God had a better plan that would demonstrate his power, rather than the people's power.

When Joshua finally gets on board, does what he's asked, and returns to Ai following God's plan, the enemy is soundly defeated. He was reminded it was a two-way agreement, and it wasn't until Joshua did what God asked that God fulfilled his promise. (Joshua 8:3-22)

Quit Wandering and Come Home

The Bible is filled with stories of men and women just like Abraham and Joshua who thought they had a better idea, a better way. Men and women who wanted to live life on their terms and not on God's terms. The story of the prodigal son is one that many can more easily relate to than that of Abraham or Joshua.

It's really the same story, but I know I can see myself as a wanderer so much more quickly than I can admit to being disobedient. It's easier for our ego to grasp the idea of wandering away rather than full-out running away in defiance.

Luke 15 outlines the story of a father with two sons. The younger son told his father he didn't want to work the family farm anymore. It was hard work. He wanted to go do his own thing and enjoy the easy life but needed his father's inheritance to be able to do that. He didn't want to be patient and wait for it, he wanted it now. See, I told you I could relate to it.

The father, while broken-hearted I'm sure, gave the son what he wanted and watched as he packed his things and left to enjoy his life. No parent wants to watch their rebellious child walk away into what the parent knows from experience is a disaster waiting for a place to happen.

The younger son gave in to his fleshly desires and lived a wild life, satisfying his every whim while spending the fortune he'd received from his father. Just when he thinks he's hit bottom, watching all his money disappear, a famine comes over the land. With no money, or means of providing for his needs, he began to starve.

In an attempt to stay alive, he started looking for work. He was able to find it working in a local farmer's field. It wasn't a noble job. After all, he was feeding the pigs on this farm. But he did what he had to do to survive.

After a time of suffering through the humility of feeding someone's pigs just to survive, he realized he hadn't ended up where he'd planned when he left his father's house. He also had set out for Seattle and ended up in Mexico. So how did he fix the problem he currently faced? What did he need to do to get back on track and end up with the "good life" he so desperately sought?

Although he didn't want to, he realized it was as simple as returning home to the loving father who so faithfully cared and provided for him. That realization couldn't have been easy.

What would his father say?

What if he was still angry over the financial loss and the pain caused him when his son left?

What if his father couldn't forgive him?

I've been there. I've come to that same realization. After suffering the shame and humiliation of the pig slop I was living in, all I wanted to do was go home where it was safe. To go where I'm loved just for who I am, not for what I can do for someone.

I've asked myself those same questions.

What if God is too angry over what I've done and the mess I've made?

What if my heavenly father can't forgive me?

Do I have what it takes to humble myself?

Do I have the strength to take that first step on the road back home?

The prodigal son did. He humbled himself before his father and confessed his sins. He acknowledged the depth of his sin, declaring, "I am no longer worthy of being called your son." (Luke 15:21)

Did his father respond with a quick retort, exclaiming, "You're right about that! What were you thinking? How could you do this to me? Seriously, what were you thinking?"

Sometimes parents respond that way when you do something stupid. That's certainly what they're thinking and sometimes it's even the first words out of their mouth. But not this father.

This father was so overjoyed his son had finally come home, he ran to meet him. His father saw him coming from a distance and couldn't contain his joy. I can just picture this lonely father sitting on the porch watching and waiting, wondering where his son might be. Wondering when his son would come home. Worried sick over what might be happening to him. Had danger come upon him? Was he safe? Was he even alive? Just watching. And waiting. Until finally, he sees him in the distance.

There were no thoughts about the money or the pain he'd suffered. He was only thinking about the joy he felt seeing his lost son returning home. He was thinking about the joy of being able to hold him again. The joy of being able to care for him again. To keep him safe from harm. To experience the joy of just sitting beside him on that porch. The joy of just looking at him and talking with him any time he wanted. The joy of watching him sleep.

God, my father, feels all these things about me. All those years, I was off on my own thinking I could handle things by myself. All those years, I lived in pig slop just trying to survive. I'm certain it was difficult for him to know I was suffering the natural consequences that followed my actions. But he waited. I'm also certain he missed me all those years I was away from home. But again, he waited.

God sat there on that porch, looking longingly into the distance, watching and waiting for me to return. There were no angry thoughts. There were no thoughts of the pain he suffered missing me while I was away. He just ached to see me again and tell me, "Quit wandering, child! Come home!"

God's Plan Finally Fulfilled for Me

My life in the pigpen is over. My plan, Plan A, didn't work out like I thought. It's time for Plan B, which is taking that first step back home. I'm ready to head back and admit what a terrible mistake I made by walking away intent on running my own life. I'm ready to admit I'm not worthy to be called daughter, ask for forgiveness, and trust my father will take me back.

Admitting I need to switch to Plan B implies the first plan didn't work. That's why I need to switch to a different plan and take another stab at it. While the first plan didn't yield the results I wanted, that doesn't mean it was a bad thing.

My Plan B might be God's Plan A. It might just be the plan he's had for me all along. While I was suffering the consequences of my poor choices and distance from God, he sat on that front porch waiting for me to make the first step back.

I'll admit, it's often hard for me to understand how God could allow all those things to happen to me if he had a better plan all along. Then I remember the words he spoke to Joshua, "Get up! Why are you lying on your face? Israel has sinned and broken my covenant. You will never defeat your enemies until you remove these things from among you." (Joshua 7:6-13) God reminds me my suffering is a result of my inability to do as he expected. Let me stop for a moment and clarify that statement before anyone misunderstands.

While the first plan didn't yield the results I wanted, that doesn't mean it was a bad thing.

I'm not suggesting my rape was a consequence for my lack of obedience. What I'm suggesting is that my poor reaction to that event and subsequent poor behavior is what resulted in all the suffering I've had over the past forty years.

I could've turned to God with my pain, trusted him to care for me and heal my hurt. It was the hours and days after my rape where I sidetracked God's Plan A. When I decided I didn't need a God who would allow this to happen, that's when God stepped aside and let me practice my free will.

Unlike those boys, God is a gentleman. He would never force himself or his plan on me. He desires more than anything for me to want him and his plan.

When I decided I no longer wanted that, I was on my own. He didn't desert me. He sat on that porch longing for me to come home where he could care for me and keep me safe.

In spite of my misunderstanding that God couldn't possibly love me or have my best interest in mind if he let this unspeakable act happen to me, I have to remember God never promised my life would be without suffering.

In fact, quite the opposite. He said "after" I suffered he would lift me up.

Until the day I realize suffering is a fact of life with Christ, I'll be alone living out my plan. God wants me to realize my Plan A isn't working and switch to Plan B, which was his plan all along.

Until I do, he'll wait patiently for me to come home. Once I let go of my past, my plans, and my sufferings and make up my mind to trust his plan, he'll rush off that porch and grab me in his embrace. Once I let go of these things, he'll bring me victory and the blessings he's been waiting so long to share with me.

Waiting or Expecting

Abraham, Joshua, and even the prodigal son waited on God. They waited for him to fix their circumstances and give them the joyful life he promised. But that's the problem. They waited.

Wait: to remain inactive or in a state of repose, as until something expected happens.[1] *To remain inactive until something happens*. Is that how I should wait for God's promises to bless me?

Obedience doesn't follow blessings; blessings follow obedience.

Even Abraham, Joshua, and the prodigal son learned the truth about that. In the end, they all learned God's covenant to bless them didn't come without some effort and sacrifice on their part.

They learned God isn't a genie who appears when we're in need, granting our every wish to make all our problems go away.

They also learned God expected them to obey first. I can only imagine God's face when he hears us say, "If you do this for me now, God, I'll do this for you later." Obedience doesn't follow blessings; blessings follow obedience.

The interesting word in the definition of wait is "expected." It says we remain inactive until something expected happens.

Expect: to look forward to; regard as likely to happen; anticipate the occurrence, or the coming of.[2] *Regard as likely to happen, anticipate the occurrence*.

If something is truly expected, if we truly anticipate it happening, do we spend our time waiting on it, remaining inactive, or do we actively prepare for it?

Let's play the word association game. What's the first word that comes to your mind when you hear the word "expecting"?

For me, it's pregnancy or baby. When I found out I was pregnant, I fully expected after nine months to walk out of that hospital with a baby. From the day the doctor announced I was pregnant, I started living every day fully expecting a baby would arrive on my delivery date. We didn't tell our friends, "We're waiting for a baby." No! We told them, "We're expecting a baby." There's a clear difference.

I didn't wait for God to change things, I prepared for when things changed.

Even when there was no way to see the baby, or understand the changes in my body, I still knew he was there. I didn't just sit around and wait for nine months, wondering, "God, when will you change my circumstances so I'm not gaining all this weight and throwing up every day?" (I'm not making that up. I literally was sick for nine months, and even vomited in the delivery room.) Okay, I'll admit it, those words probably at least crossed my mind, if not my lips, when I left the doctor's office three weeks after my due date with the reassurance my baby would come when he was ready.

During what seemed like an endless pregnancy, I didn't wait for God to change things. I prepared for when things would change. I believed 100% my son would arrive at the appointed time. I prepared a nursery. I purchased clothing, diapers, all sorts of baby gadgets and equipment.

I knew when my nine months were up, that baby would appear. After all, no woman has been pregnant forever. That thought did give me some hope in those long three weeks after my due date.

I need to live like that every day. I need to expect God to deliver on his promises. If he promised I would spend eternity with him, I should fully expect at the end of my life to spend eternity with him.

With that expectation in mind, I should prepare for the arrival of that promise. I need to start believing everything will happen in God's timing. It's not nine months like a pregnancy, thankfully, but God knows the perfect time to deliver me from this life and take me to heaven.

Job 14:5 tells me, "You have decided the length of our lives. You know how many months we will live, and we are not given a minute longer." Just like my baby. He came at the perfect time. Not when I wanted, but when God wanted.

Someone told me, as I sat there in tears three weeks overdue and fifty pounds heavier, "Wishing and wanting will not make it so!" But when I held my son in my arms, all the preparation, vomiting, and suffering was forgotten.

Although there were many times during that pregnancy when I could no longer see an end in sight, I knew there was an end coming. As storms come and go in our lives, we can count on the fact they will, eventually, come to an end.

That fact by itself won't necessarily give you peace, but knowing while you're in the storm that God is working hard to prepare the rainbow might. What also might is knowing the words of Romans 8:18: the pain you're feeling can't compare to the joy that's coming!

My pregnancy wasn't fun. Nor was it easy. Due to complications, I almost died following delivery. However, when I held my son for the first time, there was no doubt God had been working hard in the background, creating a beautiful rainbow for me that I now call Jared.

Every time I look at him and remember the joy I felt at his arrival, it gives me hope and strength to continue to believe, expect, and prepare for the promise God will bring me at the end of my life. For I know, when God's perfect time has come, and his perfect plan is complete, I'll hear that trumpet blow, I'll meet Jesus in the air, and all suffering will be forgotten! Nothing will ever be the same!

My Plan A wasn't so hot, but I think I'm going to like Plan B.

Inspiration Suggestions

> *If you return to the Almighty, you will be restored—so clean up your life. Job 22:23*

> *So he returned home to his father. And while he was still a long way off, his father saw him coming. Filled with love and compassion, he ran to his son, embraced him, and kissed him. His son said to him, 'Father, I have sinned against both heaven and you, and I am no longer worthy of being called your son.' But his father said to the servants, 'Quick! Bring the finest robe in the house and put it on him. Get a ring for his finger and sandals for his feet. And kill the calf we have been fattening. We must celebrate with a feast, for this son of mine was dead and has now*

171

returned to life. He was lost, but now he is found.' So the party began. Luke 15:20-24

➤ *To walk out of his will is to walk into nowhere. C. S. Lewis*

➤ *As you walk with Jesus, resting your head on His heart, you will learn to know His Word, His will, and His ways. You will want to obey him, not out of forced compliance, but out of heartfelt connection. Your joy will abound as you remain in His love. Sue Detweiler*

➤ *There are no secrets to success. It is the result of preparation, hard work, and learning from failure. Colin Powell*

➤ *Instead, let us test and examine our ways. Let us turn back to the Lord. Lamentations 3:40*

➤ *Song – "Prodigal" by Sidewalk Prophets**

➤ *Song – "Oh Lord" by Lauren Daigle**

*Video available at https://bit.ly/2I38TXv

Reflect

1. Do you consciously think about, plan, and live out the life you desire, or do you allow your day-to-day experiences to dictate your direction? What steps can you take to regain control?

2. Have you climbed what you thought was the ladder to success only to find it didn't lead to where you wanted to go? What can you do to reposition your ladder to ensure you get to where you want in life?

3. When things seem impossible, do you have a hard time believing in

God's promises without question? Have you ever tried to force something to happen rather than waiting on God's timing?

4. Have you been expecting to receive God's blessings without obeying the terms of your covenant with him? What are the terms? What does God expect you to do with your life?

5. Have you ever given in to your fleshly desires and lived a wild life and then after suffering the shame and humiliation that often accompanies poor choices had to ask for forgiveness?

6. Have you been waiting for God to change things or preparing for when things change? What can you do to better prepare yourself for when things change?

7. Which Inspiration Suggestions did you choose to explore, and which stood out you'd like to remember?

8. What action steps do you need to take to implement what you've discovered in this chapter?

13

I Need to Count My Blessings

Positive Self-Talk

Is the glass half-full or half-empty?
Is the grass really greener on the other side of the fence?
Does everyone else truly have it better than I do?
I actually have the answers to these age-old questions! Would you like me to share my wisdom? Here you go!

The glass is probably neither half-full nor half-empty. Statistically, it is more likely slightly above or below that exact center point.

The grass on the other side of the fence is probably not any greener unless they painted it or put in a whole lot more work than I did.

And, chances are, not many people have it any better than I do. If they do, they probably also have bigger credit card bills.

You may have noticed a trend with those answers. Everything in life is based on your perspective. I saw a graphic once that asked the question, "How high is the mud?" It showed a picture of a small dog covered in mud halfway up its belly next to a large dog whose paws were the only thing covered in mud. That really drives home the point about perspective. Two people can see the same situation quite differently.

With depression, we're prone to see the mud as halfway up our belly when the truth is, we may barely be muddy at all. Things often seem much worse than they are. I read a story once about a son asking his father how big God is. The father pointed out a plane in the sky and asked his son how big it was. The son declared it to be very small. The father then took his son to the airport where they could see planes up close. When he asked his son again how big the plane was, his son had a completely different answer. Things that are up close and personal to us seem much larger than the exact same thing from a distance. It's all about from what perspective we are viewing the problem.

Distorted Vision

Have you ever gone to the eye doctor and had him ask, "Which is better—one or two?" If not, congratulations! You obviously were gifted with great vision. I, on the other hand, have horrible vision. I've worn glasses or contacts since I was in third grade. Nothing ever seemed clear until the doctor put that machine in front of my face and started dialing in my preferences. A *one* here. A *two* there. Next thing you know, I have new glasses, and I can see everything perfectly. My eyes didn't change, my focus did.

Prior to getting those new glasses, I didn't see things as they actually were, I saw them through my distorted, unclear vision. Depression is the same way. We tend to see things through our distorted, unclear view of the world. We tend to see everything from a negative perspective.

However, it doesn't have to be that way. Just like getting glasses changed my visual focus from being distorted and unclear, a change in my mental focus can do the same for how I view my circumstances.

My eyes didn't change, my focus did. Are we back to the "just think happy thoughts" advice? No, of course not. We're at a place where we need to recognize focusing on negative thoughts is not the answer. It's not going to help our situation. Let's face it, our mind is going to focus on something. It is constantly moving and thinking. If we don't control it, it will control us.

If your mind tends to focus on the many stressful, negative circumstances in your life, it's time to start focusing on the many blessings you have in your life instead. It is possible to go from stressed to blessed by simply changing the focus of your thoughts.

Out with the Old

Our thoughts are never silent. Or at least mine aren't. The more I try to clear my mind, the more thoughts come to my mind. You know those meditation rituals that tell you to clear your mind? I haven't mastered those. What I've learned, though, is the value of replacing unproductive thoughts with productive ones.

When I was in the hospital, we went through a meditation class. They played soft music and told us to clear our mind and just focus on the music. Believe me, I tried. Although my thoughts were no longer on my troubles, they weren't gone. They had simply moved from bad thoughts about all that was wrong to thoughts of whether I liked the music, or how it made me feel, or the picture of a soothing place I thought of when I heard the music.

> *It is possible to go from stressed to blessed by simply changing the focus of your thoughts.*

But I think that's the point. My thoughts weren't silent, they had just refocused on something more productive. They had refocused on thoughts that made me feel calmer and more at peace. I was practicing a form of mind control. That's the moment I realized I get to choose which thoughts my mind will focus on.

In Toby Mac's song "Speak Life," we are reminded to think and say things that are helpful and not hurtful. Many believe that means when we speak to other people, and it does. But it also means when we speak to ourselves. I know what you're thinking—only crazy people talk to themselves. I disagree. Everyone talks to themselves. However, smart people control what they say to themselves. It's time to take back the narrative and control the conversation you have with yourself.

What do I mean? Have you ever said to yourself, either out loud or in your head, I'm so stupid, I'm so fat, or I can't ever do anything right? This is the opposite of speaking life. Your mind is very gullible, and it will believe what you tell it. The more you say these negative things, the more you'll believe they're true, that you are in fact a stupid, fat, idiot who can never do anything right.

Maybe you've made some mistakes or gained a few extra pounds. Maybe you've lost your way. Maybe you aren't the perfect person you envisioned you would be at this point in your life. However, you are a child of God made in his image. He made you just the way you are and loves the perfectly imperfect person you are.

> **You are a child of God made in his image. He made you just the way you are and loves the perfectly imperfect person you are.**

That doesn't give us license to belittle God's creation, though. God always sees the best in us and wants us to do the same. It's time to clean house and let go of all the negative thoughts we have and negative images we see of ourselves. Not just clearing your mind of them but replacing them with positive thoughts and images more in line with the way God sees you.

Many times, our past contributes to those negative thoughts and images. Although it often seems like there's no way to escape your past, I have confidence God can do it because he's done it for me. Whether the past that's plaguing you was ten minutes ago, ten weeks ago, or ten years ago, it's time to let it go. Quit looking in the rearview mirror and leave the past where it belongs—behind you. Look ahead to the promise of an abundant life, which God wants to give you.

Second Chances

That sounds wonderful, doesn't it? Forget all your past mistakes and misfortune and start fresh. Every athlete has that same dream. There was a theme song of sorts for one of the Olympics when I was younger entitled "One Moment in Time." Whitney Houston belted out the chorus, which stated the thoughts of every athlete in the games. They all want the same thing—just one moment in time to show who they really are and all they can do. However, as we discussed earlier, only one of them in each event will have the opportunity to feel that victory. All the others share one common thing outside of their win or lose status. They share the overwhelmingly strong desire for a second chance. A do-over.

The movie *The Replacements* is based on that same theme. The quarterback for this team of rag-tag players, who steps in during a strike, just wants the chance to overcome the poor reputation he earned as a player years before. Apparently, he had one of the worst games of his life in a very big and well-televised Sugar Bowl game. Everybody saw his failures and they won't quickly forgive or forget them. He wants a second chance to show the world what he can do. He wants another moment in time to show the world all that he knows he can be.

In with the New

We all feel like that. We want that second chance. It even sounds fairly simple—show the world you're not the person they think you are.

I certainly wanted a second chance to show all those people who knew me during my dark decade to see the new me. I didn't go to a high school reunion for thirty years. Once I recovered from my breakdown and had a different view of myself, I suddenly was excited to go see them all again.

Nothing had changed. I wasn't richer, thinner, or more successful. I just finally believed the truth about myself based on God's standards. For the first time, I truly felt like the daughter of the King of Kings, who was made in his image. I finally felt like someone worthy of love and respect.

While it is a simple process to replace old, negative thoughts with new, more positive ones, it's not easy to do. But it can be done. I'm living proof. It all starts with mind control.

Not the negative kind of mind control you see in movies where a really bad villain makes a really innocent victim do something they would never do if they were in control of their thoughts. The movie *Divergent* comes to mind. One of the factions is given a drug that turns them into an army forced to do the evil bidding of the person controlling their minds. These are good people who would never knowingly hurt the people they've been forced to hurt.

The same thing happens to each of us on a daily basis. Negative thoughts that can hurt us constantly attempt to take control of our mind. We have to stop them using what I call Positive Mind Control.

Positive Mind Control

Positive Mind Control is the act of constantly monitoring every thought that attempts to take up space in our mind and the removal of any thoughts that don't support the positive lifestyle you're attempting to have. It's your own personal TSA agent (like at the airport). If a negative thought or emotion tries to take hold, your Positive Mind Control (PMC) agent will assess the situation and determine whether it is a risk to your mental health. If the thought or emotion doesn't support a positive life, your PMC agent will deny it access. That way your mind is always controlled by thoughts and emotions that support the life you're trying to build.

Positive Mind Control is the act of constantly monitoring every thought that attempts to take up space in our mind and the removal of any thoughts that don't support the positive lifestyle you're attempting to have.

In 2 Corinthians 10:5, we are reminded to "take every thought captive." In the context of the surrounding verses, Paul is trying to teach the Corinthians to stop thinking from a worldly perspective and make sure all thoughts line up with God's perspective. We need to do the same.

We read another reminder about PMC in Romans 12:2, which says, "Don't copy the behavior and customs of this world, but let God transform you into a new person by changing the way you think."

I believe these verses combine very well. First, we learn to take every thought captive to make sure it aligns with God's purposes and then we allow him to change the way we think. If a thought doesn't align, he will give us a new thought to replace it—if we give him that power. But that starts with the PMC agent assessing every thought against the guidelines set out for us in Philippians 4:8: "Fix your thoughts on what is true, and honorable, and right, and pure, and lovely, and admirable."

That first test—is it true—is a hard one. That's because our truth doesn't always line up with God's truth. Let's go back to the "I'm a stupid, fat, idiot who can never do anything right" conversation. That may be your truth, but it certainly isn't God's truth. His truth is that he created you in his image and you are a child of God.

Learning to apply this first test will take some time because some of you may need to learn what God's truth about you is first. If that's you, I would start by studying God's Word regularly to get to know him and what he says about his children. If you're short on time, a good place to start would be with the list of God's attributes I outlined in Chapter 6 and the starter list of positive affirmations I've outlined below. I call it a starter list because you're going to want to add to it, subtract from it, and or modify it to best meet your needs. Memorize the ones that speak to you most. Put them on cards or sticky notes and keep them with you wherever you might need a reminder of what the truth is about who you are.

Positive Affirmations

Keep in mind that simply reciting positive affirmations will not change your life. You must be actively attempting to replace the negative thoughts and beliefs you currently hold with these newer, more positive beliefs—not simply because they are positive, but because you believe they are true.

The power is not in the words themselves, but in the ability to believe they are true of your life.

There is no power in these words. The power comes from believing them. If your mind even hints at doubt or laughs at the statement, explore why. It's that internal work that will yield results.

First, I will give you a few positive affirmations from the word of God because I believe that's where our power lies—in God's truth. Then I will give you a few from some well-known speakers on the topic, such as the king of positive affirmations, Jack Canfield. Some of them really speak to me. However, be cautious with positive affirmations from others, no matter how well-known. Again, the power is not in the words themselves, but in the ability to believe they are true of your life.

- ✓ I am strong and courageous because God is with me. Joshua 1:9

- ✓ I will stand firm when my enemies fall. Psalm 20:7-8

- ✓ I will place my hope in God. Psalm 25:5

- ✓ God's love for me never fails. Psalm 36:7

- ✓ I can trust God to do what he promised. Psalm 138:8

- ✓ God thinks about me all the time. Psalm 139:17

- ✓ I am strong and worthy of respect. Proverbs 31:25

- ✓ I will not be discouraged or afraid for God is with me. Isaiah 41:10

- ✓ I am precious to God—I am honored and loved. Isaiah 43:4

- ✓ I will forget my shame—God has redeemed me. Isaiah 54:4-6

✓ I can face anything today because God forgives my mistakes and provides comfort for my hardships before I even start my day. Lamentations 3:23

✓ I am never alone—God is always with me. Matthew 1:23

✓ I am a child of God. John 1:12-13

✓ I can endure anything because the joy of heaven far outweighs any suffering I'm experiencing right now. Romans 8:18

✓ When I face obstacles, God shows me a way out. 1 Cor 10:13

✓ I am God's masterpiece. Ephesians 2:10

✓ I have learned to be content. Philippians 4:11

✓ When I am weak, God's strength makes me strong. Philippians 4:13

✓ I have everything I need—God provides for me. Philippians 4:19

✓ I have been rescued from the darkness. Colossians 1:13

✓ I will not panic—God gave me a calm, peaceful mind. 2 Tim 1:7

✓ I have real contentment and feel truly safe because I trust in God not in things. Hebrews 13:6

✓ When I suffer, God will restore me and make me even better than before. 1 Peter 5:10

✓ I can conquer the world when Christ lives in me. 1 John 4:4

✓ God keeps me safe—Satan can't touch me. 1 John 5:18

✓ All that I seek is already within me. Jack Canfield

✓ I am focused and persistent. I will never quit. Jack Canfield

✓ I believe in myself and my ability to succeed. Jack Canfield

✓ I am in the process of positive change. Jack Canfield

✓ I am continually clearing out old things in my life to make space for the new things I want. Jack Canfield

✓ My past is not a reflection of my future. Unknown

✓ I have the power to create change. Jennifer Kass

✓ I can. I will. End of Story. Unknown

Inspiration Suggestions

➢ *Affirmations are our mental vitamins, providing the supplementary positive thoughts we need to balance the barrage of negative events and thoughts we experience daily. Tia Walker*

➢ *The biggest obstacle you'll ever have to overcome is your mind. If you can overcome that, you can overcome anything. Marc Chernoff*

➢ *Truth be told, it never pays to get discouraged. Staying mindful and making positivity a way of life will help you restore your faith in yourself, no matter what you're up against. Marc Chernoff*

➢ *Being positive doesn't mean ignoring the negative. Being positive means overcoming the negative. There's a big difference between the two. Marc Chernoff*

➢ *Once you replace negative thoughts with positive ones, you'll start having positive results. Willie Nelson*

➢ *The greatest discovery of all time is that a person can change his future by merely changing his attitude. Oprah Winfrey*

➢ *A negative mind will never give you a positive life. Ziad K. Abdelnour*

➢ *Song – "One Moment in Time" by Whitney Houston**

➤ *Song – "Old Church Choir" by Zach Williams**

➤ *Song – "Speak Life" by Toby Mac**

*Video available at https://bit.ly/2I38TXv

Reflect

1. Have you ever had the opportunity to see an object or situation from two different perspectives? How did it change your view of it?

2. If you're honest with yourself, would you say you tend to see things more from the negative (glass half-empty) or positive (glass half-full) perspective? Why?

3. How has your perspective affected your thoughts and emotions?

4. Do you have trouble clearing your mind or controlling your thoughts? What steps can you take to stop negative thoughts before they take hold in your mind and replace them with positive thoughts that are more productive?

5. Do you tend to obsess over negative experiences by replaying negative situations over and over in your mind while downplaying or ignoring positive situations? What can you do to stop this destructive habit?

6. Do you want a do-over—a second chance? Why? What do you want to change? How would this change make things better?

7. How do you want people to see you differently? More importantly, how do you need to see yourself differently?

8. Do you need to hire a PMC agent? What are the top five negative thoughts you need to place on your no-fly list? Why do they need to be there and how will eliminating them help?

9. Pick five positive affirmations from the list that, if you memorized them and spoke them out loud to yourself at least once every day, would begin to make a positive impact on your mind.

10. Which Inspiration Suggestions did you choose to explore, and which stood out you'd like to remember?

11. What action steps do you need to take to implement what you've discovered in this chapter?

PART
IV

How Do I Help Others?

14

I Need to Help Others

The Voice of Experience

They're all around us. In our homes. On our bus. At our school. In our office. They're even at our church. What do they look like? They're short, tall, fat, thin, black, white, young, and old. They're taking over the world. Who are they? Hurting people! There's a saying that hurting people hurt people. If that's true, we've got to do something quick because we don't need more hurting people in our world. But how can we help?

Don't Just Walk By

The first step is to become more aware of how many people around us are struggling. According to the National Alliance on Mental Illness,

> "Depression is a common illness, affecting more than 350 million people of all ages around the world. It's currently the number one cause of disability, and is predicted to be the number one global burden of disease by 2030."[1]

The National Alliance on Mental Illness goes on to tell us one in five adults experience a mental illness each year, and over 17 million adults in the United States alone suffered at least one major depressive episode in 2018.

That's about 7% of all U.S. adults."[2] Assuming that's true, that means most likely several of your closest family and friends is struggling with depression.

Does that surprise you? Did you think you were the only one? It's not uncommon to feel alone and isolated in your depression. Most people with depression feel like no one else could possibly understand what they're going through. However, that's simply not true.

Take a minute to make a list of your ten closest family members or friends. Now, scan down your list. Can you pick out who might be struggling based on those statistics? Have there been signs before now that you missed? This question has caused me a lot of anguish over the past few weeks as I've lost two people in my so-called sphere of influence to suicide.

At a time like this you ask yourself how you could have missed it. And worse yet, if you saw the signs and didn't do anything, why not? What were you afraid of? Let me stop here to clarify something before I trigger something painful in someone.

Let me say it loud and clear—it is not anyone else's fault when someone chooses to take their own life. You can't stop people from doing something they're hell-bent on doing. Let's go back to what we learned earlier—you can't control people, places, things, or events.

In the two cases I mentioned, like in the majority of others, multiple attempts were made by different people to help the hurting person but to no avail. Also, helping someone in that frame of mind is a job best left to the professionals. The best thing you can do is to point them in the direction of a mental health professional and encourage them to go. Make an emergency referral if it's appropriate. Then keep an eye on them and pray.

It is not anyone else's fault when someone chooses to take their own life. You can't stop people from doing something they're hell-bent on doing.

With that said, there are many people around you right now who are hurting. They feel alone and don't think anyone else will understand what they're going through. Sound familiar? We've all been there.

These hurting people are currently walking down a road you and I have already been down. And even though you see them regularly, you may not notice them or their struggle. It's a common mistake. Our focus is on our own lives and the activities we're engaged in. For the most part, we walk through life with blinders on. But it's time to open our eyes and see those in our path who may need help.

The Lame Beggar

A perfect example is the story of the lame beggar sitting at the temple gate in Acts 3. The man sat at the Beautiful Gate every day in order to beg for money as the people entered the temple. Seems like a great plan. After all, people came to the temple several times a day to pray. Good people. Faithful people. People who supposedly believed what the scriptures taught them about caring for others.

Unfortunately, things didn't quite work out according to his plan. These so-called caring citizens of Jerusalem walked right past him on their way into and out of the temple. They walked past him, but they didn't see him. They became so desensitized to his presence that they no longer saw his need.

Peter and John saw the lame beggar, though. They saw him and his need, and they knew they had something that could help end his suffering.

We need to stop being like the Roman citizens walking right past hurting people, oblivious to their needs. We need to stop focusing on our own lives long enough to see the pain in those around us. And once we see it, we need to understand we have something that might help.

Even if it's just a shoulder to cry on, an ear to listen, or someone to sit with them quietly so they don't feel so alone. Don't forget, you've been there. You know what helped you or at least what would have helped if someone had offered. Be that light in the darkness for someone else.

The Good Samaritan

Another more well-known example is the story of the good Samaritan in Luke 10:25-37. A man was robbed, beaten, and left for dead on a well-traveled desert road between Jericho and Jerusalem. Several people walked right past the hurting man. They saw him, but didn't see or, worse yet, didn't care about his need. They even went so far as to walk by on the other side of the road. They not only didn't want to help him, they wanted to avoid him. It wasn't for a lack of time or ability to help; it was through an apathetic and selfish attitude. They simply didn't want to be bothered. They had their own problems to deal with. They had their own places to go and people to see. But don't we all?

That's a serious problem in our society. For the most part, we're all too self-absorbed to help others in need. We're so busy seeing all our own problems, we don't have time or energy to see those of others. It's time to break that cycle of disinterest in the needs of others.

Now that we know the life or death battle the fight with depression can be, how can we turn a blind eye to someone who is suffering? The Samaritan man decided he couldn't ignore the hurting man in front of him. He couldn't just walk by and ignore him. He needed to help him. He set the example for us to follow.

Make a Difference

Can we help them all? Of course not! That's why one of my favorite poems is *The Star Thrower* (aka Starfish Poem). It points out the futility thinking of so many. If I can't help them all, why bother? Because each and every person struggling is worth saving! You can make a difference for that one!

You're absolutely right about not being able to save the world. Good news though—that's not your job! However, you can offer support to a person who's struggling. If they choose to accept it, you've made a difference that could save one life from suffering a single day longer than necessary. You can learn to be compassionate. According to Compassion International, the meaning of compassion is to recognize the suffering of others, then take action to help. They go on to say it's so much more than simply feelings of empathy or care. Based on the Latin roots of the word, the meaning of compassion is to "suffer with."[3]

After my breakdown, I believe I was called to use my suffering to help others. To suffer with them. In fact, I believe we're all called to use our suffering to help others. Don't you wish someone had been there to help you? If someone was there for you, do you wish they'd been there sooner? You can be that person for someone else.

Now It's My Turn

When I first started sharing my story, a close friend said, "You give me the confidence and courage to face my own issues." That's what sharing your

The Star Thrower

"Once upon a time, there was a wise man who used to go to the ocean to do his writing. He had a habit of walking on the beach before he began his work.

One day, as he was walking along the shore, he looked down the beach and saw a human figure moving like a dancer. He smiled to himself at the thought of someone who would dance to the day, and so, he walked faster to catch up.

As he got closer, he noticed that the figure was that of a young man, and that what he was doing was not dancing at all. The young man was reaching down to the shore, picking up small objects, and throwing them into the ocean.

He came closer still and called out "Good morning! May I ask what it is that you are doing?"

The young man paused, looked up, and replied, "Throwing starfish into the ocean."

"I must ask, then, why are you throwing starfish into the ocean?" asked the somewhat startled wise man.

To this, the young man replied, "The sun is up and the tide is going out. If I don't throw them in, they'll die."

Upon hearing this, the wise man commented, "But, young man, do you not realize that there are miles and miles of beach and there are starfish all along every mile? You can't possibly make a difference!"

At this, the young man bent down, picked up yet another starfish, and threw it into the ocean. As it met the water, he said, "It made a difference for that one."

Loren Eiseley

story can do for someone you know. Someone has to step out and be the first. Why not let it be you?

Now, you may not be ready to share your story and your pain in a public forum like I have. That's okay. Not everyone is. Some never will be. However, you can sit down one-on-one with a close friend or family member and sincerely say, "I genuinely do understand what you're going through because I've been right where you are now." Then share a little about your own struggle. The conversation will flow naturally from there as a huge weight will most likely be lifted off the one with whom you're sharing.

The words of the song "The Words I Would Say" by Sidewalk Prophets sums it up best. That song was one of my main inspirations to write this book. It basically asks you to ponder this thought—if you know someone is struggling with something you've already learned how to conquer, what would you want them to know? What words could you say to help them conquer their own problems?

Now that you recognize you have a way to help others, can you honestly sit back and not take action? Can you continue to walk past those suffering friends and family members without offering them the support they need? The best support you can offer them is the voice of experience! Don't keep it to yourself!

Inspiration Suggestions

➢ *I don't want to live in the kind of world where we don't look out for each other. Not just the people that are close to us, but anybody who needs a helping hand. I can't change the way anybody else thinks, or what they choose to do, but I can do my bit. Charles DeLint*

➢ *One of the most important things you can do on this earth is to let people know they are not alone. Shannon L. Adler*

➢ *It's not enough to have lived. We should be determined to live for something. May I suggest that it be creating joy for others, sharing what we have for the betterment of personkind, bringing hope to the lost and love to the lonely. Leo Buscaglia*

➢ *Carry each other's burdens, and in this way you will fulfill the law of Christ. Galatians 6:2*

➢ *Song – "Hope in Front of Me" by Danny Gokey**

➢ *Song – "Warrior" by Hannah Kerr**

➢ *Song – "Words I Would Say" by Sidewalk Prophets**

➢ *Song – "Does Anybody Hear Her" by Casting Crowns**

➢ *Song – "Give Me Your Eyes" by Brandon Heath**

➢ **Video available at https://bit.ly/2I38TXv*

Reflect

1. Who are the people on your list who may be struggling with depression? What signs have you seen that make you think that?

2. What kind of help do you wish you had received when you were struggling with depression?

3. How could you provide that same help for someone else?

4. What are the words you would to say to someone with depression?

5. How can you talk with someone who is struggling with depression? Think of each person on your list and make a plan for how you might go about starting a conversation with them about their depression.

6. Which Inspiration Suggestions did you choose to explore, and which stood out you'd like to remember?

7. What action steps do you need to take to implement what you've discovered in this chapter?

15

I Need to Change My Focus

Looking Ahead and Not Behind

You've been hanging on to the tree for dear life. The raging floodwaters rush around you and try to pull you back in. Your fingers are numb from the cold and ripped open from the struggle. You don't know how much longer you can hold on. Yet holding on brings safety.

As long as you hold on, the floodwaters can't pull you back under or slam you against the rocks or ram you into that rooftop now just barely above the surface of the water. Letting go is certain death.

Or is it?

You constantly scan the skies for a rescue helicopter because you know if it can get to you, it will take you to safety. It will take you away from all this. When the helicopter finally does arrive, the rescue worker is lowered down to you. He reaches out his hand and assures you he is there to help you. He promises he will take you to safety. All you have to do is let go of the tree; let go of what you know with every fiber of your being is safe. Even though letting go means risking your life, you must trust that the hand reaching out to you really wants to save you; that voice calling out to trust him is your only true safety. All you have to do is let go.

Stepping Out of the Boat

Letting go isn't easy, especially when you're clinging to something you've convinced yourself is safe. It took me forty years to create a life that felt safe. I had put up defense systems I thought would keep me safe. But would they?

I never sat with my back to the door, because I needed to be able to see who was coming at me and know what path to take to my exit should I need it quickly. I never allowed myself to be alone with anyone I didn't know well enough to trust with my life. I never went into an elevator if there was just a single male in there. I couldn't get a massage for about thirty of those forty years for fear of anyone touching me in a secluded environment. In fact, true confession time—I brought a friend along to sit in the room with me when I got my first massage. Weird, I know.

I never allowed housekeeping to enter my hotel room if I was on a trip alone. And probably the most important defensive mechanism I set up was never talking about my past because people might not like me anymore if they knew about my dark decade.

My life was as safe as I could get. Yet even with all those safeguards in place, I still had times when I just wasn't sure. Then one day it hit me. The phrase "safe life" is kind of an oxymoron. Are we ever truly safe?

Plain and simple, life has risks. If you want to have relationships with people and interact with others, at some point you have to take a chance. You can't cling to the relative safety of the life you've created forever. As the saying goes, if you want to walk on water, you have to get out of the boat.

That saying refers to the story of Peter leaving his fishing boat to go meet Jesus when he saw him walking on water in Matthew 14:22-33. He had to decide if the joy of meeting Jesus out on the sea was greater than the fear of drowning. The first step towards experiencing the joy Jesus wanted to give him was to step out of the boat. Could you do it? A better question might be *can* you do it? True safety and the chance at new life are finally within your reach. The safety and joy you can only experience through Jesus await you if you're willing to take a step in that direction.

No More Looking Behind

Many times, we aren't willing to let go of that tree to grab the rescue worker's hand. Or we're not willing to step out of the boat to experience the joy Jesus offers. Why are we unable to take those risks? What information are we using to come to those decisions?

For most people who suffer with depression, the answer to those questions is the past. Our past has such a hold on us that it rules every decision we make, whether we realize it or not. We've subconsciously decided that our past defines who we are and will be for the rest of our lives. Our past often determines what chances we're willing to take. But as I've said before, we need to focus on the huge windshield of possibility ahead of us rather than the small rearview mirror glimpse of where we've been.

For one thing, we're not there anymore. The only value in looking back on your life is to see how far you've come. I often look back now because I'm in a healthy place. I see memories pop up on Facebook from the time when I had my breakdown and I honestly have a hard time believing that was me. Rather than make me sad, it fills me with hope to see how far I've come. It fills me with joy to see what an amazing life God has helped me build since then.

God makes his feelings very clear on this in Isaiah 43:18-19, where he says, "Forget the former things; do not dwell on the past. See, I am doing a new thing! Now it springs up; do you not perceive it? I am making a way in the wilderness and streams in the wasteland." (NIV) He wants us to forget what's happened before and focus on the new thing he wants to do in our life.

The only value in looking back on your life is to see how far you've come.

He says it again in Philippians 3:13-14: "No, dear brothers and sisters, I have not achieved it, but I focus on this one thing: Forgetting the past and looking forward to what lies ahead, I press on to reach the end of the race and receive the heavenly prize for which God, through Christ Jesus, is calling us." (NIV) Here, he's reminding us to keep our focus not on the temporary fun and problems we encounter in our everyday lives, but on the more important goal of serving God in our daily lives in a way that leads to our ultimate prize in heaven.

Our life cannot be lived in the past. The past is gone. It's over. It can't be changed no matter how badly we want it to be. Our life has to be lived in today and all the tomorrows that make up our future. Whatever problems we experienced in the past or mistakes we made yesterday are over. They can't be changed.

We can attempt to run away from them or to build a defense system against them, hurting us further, but neither of those choices will lead to the joyful life God intends for us to have. Besides, both of those options will move us even farther away from all those who love us and from the help we need.

We can't run away from God or build a defense system that he can't break through. God provides the only true path to recovery.

Jesus Provided a Way Out

My recovery journey started with the admission that I had truly made a mess of my life. I didn't start it. My rapists started it. But I jumped on board the crazy train and ran it as long as I could.

I had the choice to turn to God on that scary night. I chose not to.

I had the choice to seek help from others. I chose not to do that either.

Instead of doing either of those things, I chose to go it alone. I chose to turn away from God, the only true source of help I had available, and live my life on my terms. That is called sin.

We can't run away from God or build a defense system which he can't break through. God provides the only true path to recovery.

The best way I can describe sin to you is in terms of what I know best, which is teaching computer skills. When I started teaching many years ago, I taught typing on a typewriter. When my students would make a mistake, they would use the correction ribbon on the typewriter to correct it. They'd hit the correction key and the typewriter would go backwards over the error and place a white typed letter over the previously typed black letter. Once it had typed white over all the letters in error, they would go back and type the correct letters in black type again.

Later on, with the invention of Wite-Out®, my students would open the bottle, pull out that little brush, and paint over their mistake. Then they would blow with all their might until it dried so they could make the correction over the top.

The problem with both of these methods of correcting errors is that when I would hold their paper up to the light, I could easily see where they had made mistakes.

Eventually, I had the opportunity to teach typing on computers. What a glorious day it was for my students when they realized they could make mistakes, as students learning to type tend to do, and I would never know it.

When they printed out their paper, you could not tell the letters that had been typed correctly the first time from the letters they had corrected.

The world views sin like those students using a typewriter. When they look at us, they can easily see our sin. God on the other hand, sees sin more like those students using a computer. When he looks at us and holds us up to the light, all he sees is a perfect paper with no mistakes. Do you know why?

Colossians 1:21-22 tells us: "Once you were alienated from God and were enemies in your minds because of your evil behavior. But now he has reconciled you by Christ's physical body through death to present you holy in his sight, without blemish and free from accusation." (NIV)

When I was living in my dark decade, and for years after that when I didn't trust God enough to surrender control of my life back to him, I was alienated from God. We were enemies because of my evil behavior. The Bible tells us God cannot look on sin, and I was setting a new world's record in sinning. But God made a way. He provided Jesus as a way out. Jesus loved me enough to die on the cross to pay for my sin. I have been reconciled back to God. He sees me as blameless. He sees me like that beautiful error-free printout from the computer.

Now, Jesus did this for me centuries before my dark decade ever started. So why was I still separated from him? Do you remember what I said I did on that fateful night? I said I chose to turn from God. He didn't turn from me. I turned from him. Unfortunately, that means the depression I then suffered for the next forty years was a tragedy of my own making.

Light at the End of the Tunnel

I didn't have to live in depression all those years. God already saw me as blameless. He saw me as his perfect creation. I'm the one who had the problem. I saw myself as damaged goods. I saw myself as unworthy of his love. I'm the one that walked into that deep, dark cave and tried to live life without him.

Life with depression is like that. It often feels like you're living in a cave, where there's no light and no hope for a future. Sometimes you see a flicker of light. Something happens that makes you

God made a way. He provided Jesus as a way out. Jesus loved me enough to die on the cross to pay for my sin. I have been reconciled back to God. He sees me as blameless.

feel like maybe you can find your way out. But you don't. You may even turn around and take a step or two back towards the front of the cave. When light doesn't appear within a few steps, though, you give up and keep walking deeper and deeper into the cave, hoping beyond hope there's a way out ahead.

The light up ahead is the glorious new life he wants to give us. It's waiting up around that next curve. We just have to hang on and keep moving. We'll get there.

What you don't realize is that you're not living in a cave. You're living in a tunnel. A cave has a beginning that's light and bright, but the farther you walk into it, the darker it gets. And there's no hope of it ever getting any brighter. You're literally at a dead end.

A tunnel, on the other hand, has a beginning and an end, both of which are light and bright. The middle may be dark and scary, but there is a way out if you just keep moving. When you're walking in that tunnel, eventually you truly will see the light up ahead. It's just around the next curve.

Many people who suffer from depression would tell you not to get too excited about that light up ahead. It's not really the end of the tunnel. It's just another train coming to run you over. That's not the case when God is with us in that tunnel, though. The light up ahead is the glorious new life he wants to give us. It's waiting up around that next curve. We just have to hang on and keep moving. We'll get there.

Accepting His Solution Brings Peace

One of my favorite songs is "Hope In Front of Me" by Danny Gokey. You probably already figured that out since it's been one of my inspiration suggestions in a couple of chapters. The official video for this song shows people carrying around labels. Some they may have gotten from others, but I believe most put the label on themselves.

That's the work of Satan. He's the one who tells us we're a victim. He's the one who tells us we're unworthy. He's the one who convinces us no one will want us. That's often where depression begins.

But we don't have to believe those lies. As the video depicts, we can toss those labels into the fire and leave them behind. The words of the song remind us that there's always hope in front of us. Even when we're in the darkest part of the tunnel and we can't see it, it's still there. Even when we have a hard time believing God would want us with all the mistakes and sin in our life, there's still hope. God is still holding our hand and leading us around that curve towards the light. Towards the joyful life he has waiting for us just outside that tunnel.

During those times when we question what we believe, we need to remember Satan's lies cannot stand up to God's truth.

When Satan says I'm worthless, God says I'm a masterpiece. (Ephesians 2:10)

When Satan says I'm unlovable, God says I am so loved that he gave up his only son to die for me. (John 3:16)

When Satan says I'm all alone, God says he will go with me and never leave me. (Deuteronomy 31:6)

When Satan says I'm not good enough, God says I don't have to be. Jesus died in my place for my sin, and he IS good enough! (Hebrews 10:14)

Who are you going to believe, Satan or God? Unfortunately, I believed Satan for forty years. That was a mistake. A huge one. Don't make the same mistake I did. Choose today to believe God. Believe what he says is true, even if it goes against everything you've

> *I believe you are stronger than your struggles. I believe you will overcome your obstacles. I believe if you make an effort rather than an excuse, things will change. And most importantly, I believe you can and will find joy if you will hold on to the hope of the abundant life God has promised.*

believed for your entire life. Let's face it, what you've been believing hasn't gotten you all that far towards a joy-filled life or you wouldn't be reading this book. Why not try it God's way?

If you have trouble believing it, borrow my belief until you can. I believe you are stronger than your struggles. I believe you will overcome your obstacles. I believe if you make an effort rather than an excuse, things will change. And most importantly, I believe you can and will find joy if you will hold on to the hope of the abundant life God has promised.

I Have Decided! Will You?

You can't go back and erase or rewrite your history. However, you can write a new story from here by allowing God to help you process your past differently so you can live in victory over it. Like I am.

Recently, I was explaining to someone that I was in the process of finishing this book. She indicated she didn't realize I was an author and asked what I wrote about. I told her I wrote about overcoming depression and finding joy. She said, "So how do you do that?"

My answer was simple. Think you know what it is after spending so many hours of your life reading this book? My answer was simply this—total surrender to God.

For the forty years I struggled with depression, I trusted only in myself. I became a people pleaser addicted to attention and approval. And looking for it in all the wrong places, if you'll recall.

I became a perfectionist in an effort to prove I had some value, some worth.

I became a control freak under the mistaken assumption that I could keep myself safe if I could just control everything. Spoiler alert—I can't.

But God tells us in John 8:12, "I am the light of the world. If you follow me, you won't have to walk in darkness, because you will have the light that leads to life." I don't want to walk in darkness anymore. I don't want to live in a deep, dark cave. I want to walk in the light and in joy. So for those reasons, I have chosen to follow Jesus. Will you?

What Happened to Helping Others

You may be asking yourself what all this surrender stuff has to do with helping others. It sounds more like something I'm doing to help me, not to help others. I thought this last part of the book was about helping others now that I'm better. What gives?

Have you ever flown on an airplane? Do you actually listen to the safety briefing or are you one of those that avoids eye contact and tries to read or sleep during those? What does the flight attendant tell you to do in the case of an emergency? She tells you to place the mask on yourself before attempting to help someone else.

You matter. Your mental health matters. It's important that you are whole before you try to help someone else with their brokenness.

See any connection between the safety briefing and my talk on surrender? You have to make sure you are ok before you help someone else. If you try to help someone else get their oxygen mask on and you aren't wearing one, you will quickly run out of oxygen yourself, rendering you useless to the person you're trying to help.

The same holds true with trying to help someone else with depression. If you haven't taken the necessary time and steps to fully heal yourself, you may render yourself useless to them in their struggles. You matter. Your mental health matters. It's important that you are whole before you try to help someone else with their brokenness.

The Journey to Joy

During those dark years, God was taking all the broken pieces of my life, gathering them together, and tucking them away with the utmost of care until the time was right to repair the broken vessel I had become. Like the Japanese process known as kintsukuroi, where resin is mixed with gold or silver in order to repair cracked pottery, God makes me even more beautiful than before.[1]

The time finally came on that day in the hospital when I sat on the bed and told God I didn't want to live like that anymore. I told him if he wanted me to keep living, he'd have to do all the work. That's the day I truly surrendered my life to his control.

It's been a journey since then. I have days where surrendering is easy. Then I have days where I slip back into control mode and try to make decisions on my own. Thankfully, I've learned to avoid those days.

The journey to joy is not an easy one. It takes every fiber of your being to truly surrender every second of every day to God. I don't know of any other way to do it. But don't misunderstand what I'm saying. The doctors and medication played a huge role. However, they have no power to heal that wasn't given them by God.

True peace comes from relieving yourself of the responsibility for making everything work out right. It comes from releasing the need to control people, places, things, and events over which you had no control to begin with. It comes from keeping your thoughts in the moment. And true peace comes from taking every thought captive and forcing it to be screened by your Positive Mind Control agent to see if it's one that is safe to travel with on your journey. Those things will bring you true peace. And it's only when you've mastered the art of true peace that you will find the joy you seek.

As I sat finishing the last few words of this five-year long writing journey, I realized there was a song that summed it up quite well. Since my journey started with the song "Words I Would Say," which encouraged me to write what I wanted to say to someone suffering with depression, I think it's only appropriate to end with a song. There are so many I could choose. However, I believe the perfect one is "Scars" by I Am They. It reminds me why I am so very thankful for the scars. Not only my own personal scars, but the scars of Jesus, who suffered and died for me. Without my scars, I would never be able to appreciate the true joy that comes with victory over depression. Let me leave you with my life verse. Hopefully it will become yours as well.

1 Peter 5:6-10 – If you will humble yourselves under the mighty hand of God, in his good time he will lift you up. Let him have all your worries and cares, for he is always thinking about you and watching everything that concerns you. Be careful—watch out for attacks from Satan, your great enemy. He prowls around like a hungry, roaring lion, looking for some victim to tear apart. Stand firm when he attacks. Trust the Lord; and remember that other Christians all around the world are going through these sufferings too. After you have suffered a little while, our God, who is full of kindness through Christ, will give you his eternal glory. He personally will come and pick you up, and set you firmly in place, and make you stronger than ever. (TLB)

Inspiration Suggestions

➢ *Song – "Scars" by I Am They**

➢ *Song – "I Surrender All (All to Jesus)" by Casting Crowns**

➢ *Song – "Haven't Seen It Yet" by Danny Gokey**

➢ *Song – "Ain't No Grave" by Bethel Music**

*Video available at https://bit.ly/2I38TXv

Reflect

1. Are you holding on to the life you've created even if you're miserable? Why are you afraid to let go and see if there might be a better life out there?

2. What safeguards have you put in place to keep others from hurting you? What are you missing out on because of them?

3. Have you limited your relationships and social interactions because you are afraid to take risks with your emotions? Why are you afraid? How could you start putting yourself out there more often?

4. On an average day, how much time do you spend looking back at what has been versus looking forward at what could be? How would your life change if you could stop that destructive habit?

5. Do you view your life from the typewriter perspective or the computer printout perspective? What could you do to change that view if it's an issue for you?

6. What labels have you placed on yourself that you now realize are lies from Satan? What steps would you need to take to overcome these labels and start believing God's truth?

7. Do you believe you are stronger than your struggles? Do you believe you will overcome your obstacles? Do you believe if you made an effort rather than an excuse thing would change? Do you believe you can and will find joy? If you don't believe these things, why not?

8. If you haven't already done so, are you willing to totally surrender control of your life to Jesus? Why or why not? If not, where are you placing your trust for the power to overcome your depression?

9. If you've already surrendered to Jesus in the past but now find yourself having trouble trusting him, what can you do to surrender control again?

10. In what ways would you like to support and help others with depression once you're strong enough to do so?

11. Which Inspiration Suggestions did you choose to explore, and which stood out you'd like to remember?

12. What action steps do you need to take to implement what you've discovered in this chapter?

Note: If you indicated you would like to surrender control to Jesus to help you overcome your depression, please email me at vicki@sadnesstojoy.com so we can connect and I can help support you in that effort.

Notes

Chapter 1: I (Don't) Need to Stay Where It's Safe

1. "Tensile Strength," The Free Dictionary by Farlex, accessed May 3, 2015, http://thefreedictionary.com/tensile+strength.

2. "Experience is the Best Teacher," The Free Dictionary by Farlex, accessed May 3, 2015, https://idioms.thefreedictionary.com/experience+is+the+best+teacher.

3. "All That Glitters is Not Gold," The Free Dictionary by Farlex, accessed May 3, 2015, https://idioms.thefreedictionary.com/all+that+glitters+is+not+gold.

4. "Grass is Always Greener," The Free Dictionary by Farlex, accessed May 3, 2015, https://idioms.thefreedictionary.com/grass+is+always+greener.

5. "J.R.R Tolkien Quotes," Goodreads, accessed May 4, 2015, https://www.goodreads.com/quotes/229-all-that-is-gold-does-not-glitter-not-all-those.

Chapter 3 – I (Don't) Need to Do Everything Right

1. "The Race," Holy Joe, accessed May 6, 2015, http://holyjoe.org/poetry/anon3.htm.

Chapter 4 – I (Don't) Need to Be in Control

1. Tom Rath, *Strengths Finder 2.0*, (New York: Gallup Press, 2013).

Chapter 7 – I Need to Ask Those Who Know

1. Depression: What Is It? (2015). *Cigna Well Aware for Better Health: Your Depression Workbook*. Easton, PA.
2. Depression: What Is It? (2015). *Cigna Well Aware for Better Health: Your Depression Workbook*. Easton, PA.

Chapter 10 – I Need to Learn to Breathe

1. "Automatic Thoughts," The Free Dictionary by Farlex, accessed June 6, 2015, https://medical-dictionary.thefreedictionary.com/automatic+thoughts.

Chapter 12 – I Need a New Direction

1. "Wait," The Free Dictionary by Farlex, accessed February 10, 2016, https://www.thefreedictionary.com/wait.

2. "Expect," The Free Dictionary by Farlex, accessed February 10, 2016, https://www.thefreedictionary.com/expect.

Chapter 14 – I Need to Help Others

1. "Let's Talk About Depression," National Alliance on Mental Illness, accessed October 15, 2019, https://www.nami.org/Blogs/NAMI-Blog/January-2018/Let-s-Talk-About-Depression.

2. "Mental Health By the Numbers," National Alliance on Mental Illness, accessed November 2, 2019, https://www.nami.org/Learn-More/Mental-Health-By-the-Numbers.

3. "We Are Suffering With Children in Need," Compassion International, accessed May 1, 2019, https://www.compassion.com/about/what-is-compassion.htm.

Chapter 15 – I Need to Change My Focus

1. "What Japanese Pottery Can Teach Us About Feeling Flawed," National Alliance on Mental Illness, accessed October 15, 2019, https://www.becomingwhoyouare.net/blog/japanese-pottery-can-teach-us-feeling-flawed.

Who Am I

I am Human – I make mistakes!
I will accept my mistakes as normal, and
I will focus on my successes, not my failures.

I am Human – I have emotions!
I will experience my emotions, and
I will use self-control in order to respond to facts, not feelings!

I am Human – I have a history!
I will accept both good and bad experiences, and
I will cherish my blessings while using what I learned to help others!

I am Human – I have physical flaws!
I will accept what I see in the mirror as a unique creation, and
I will focus on what I can do instead of what I cannot do.

I am Human – I have strengths and weaknesses!
I will acknowledge I was not made to do everything perfectly, and
I will find ways to use my strengths, while seeking help for my weaknesses.

I am Human – I have unique interests and passions!
I will set aside the expectations of others, and
I will follow my heart, allowing myself to do what brings me joy.

I am Human – I understand right and wrong!
I will do what is right just because it is right, and
I will boldly speak the truth in love to myself, and others, when it is wrong.

I am Human – I am made in the image of God!
I will believe I am a masterpiece, and
I will declare I have a purpose – I am wanted – I am loved!

Vicki Huffman
Copyright © 2015

About the Author

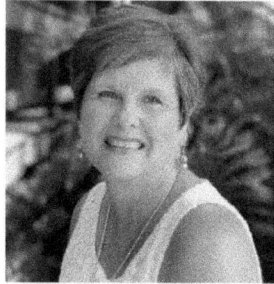

Vicki Huffman is the happily married mother of four children, two natural-born and two God entrusted her to raise for others. She is also the proud grandmother of eight. She lives in sunny Florida and lives a truly joy-filled life. However, it hasn't always been that way.

At fourteen, Vicki was the victim of a violent crime. As a result, she walked away from the God she thought would keep her safe and the faith she'd known her entire life. She wandered through life in a highly functional depressed state for the next forty years. Until that day!

On October 29, 2014, Vicki suffered a complete emotional breakdown and was hospitalized. She finally admitted she was powerless over her mental illness. She needed help. Following weeks of inpatient and outpatient care, she dedicated her time and energy to starting a new life. A joy-filled life without depression.

Vicki has learned how to leave her life of depression behind and experience a life filled with joy. As a lifelong educator, she knows her purpose in life now is to help teach those who are hurting how they too can leave depression behind and lead a joy-filled life.

To inquire about having Vicki speak at your event,
visit https://sadnesstojoy.com/speaking

Also by Vicki Huffman

21 Days to a Joy-Filled Life

Joy Journal: Creating the Life You've Always Wanted

Follow: @vickihuffman23
Questions: Email vicki@sadnesstojoy.com

21 Days to a Joy-Filled Life

The Donut Dare: Focus on All You Have,
Not All That's Missing

Vicki Huffman
Sadness to Joy Ministries

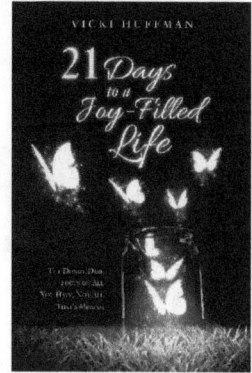

Joy is a condition many seek, but few find. On this 21-day journey, you will learn to focus on the four areas of wellness needed to live a joy-filled life: Mental, Emotional, Physical, and Spiritual.

Vicki Huffman shares how she overcame forty years of depression followed by an emotional breakdown. This is the journey to wellness she took, which led to the joy-filled life she lives today. As a lifelong educator, she understands the importance of practical application and employs it to share her success with others and lead them on the same journey.

Through daily self-assessment and habit-building activities, followed by self-reflection and adjustment, Vicki will teach you how to:

- Identify Emotional Stressors and Triggers

- Master Your Thoughts and Emotions

- Learn How Food Affects Your Mood

- Increase Face Time and Be More Spontaneous

- Regain Lost Energy and Interest in Activities

- Build a Life-Sustaining Faith

- Create Wellness Habits

Throughout this 21-day journey, Vicki will help you create your own personal Wellness Action Plan and develop a Wellness Toolkit designed to master these areas, and more, leading to less stress and more joy in your life.

Joy Journal

Creating the Life You've Always Wanted

Vicki Huffman
Sadness to Joy Ministries

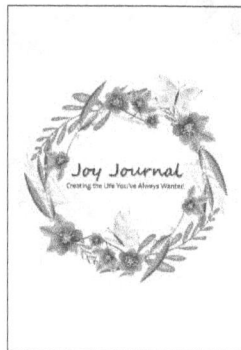

Are you living your dream life?

For most people, the answer would be a resounding no. We want to be thinner, fitter, more fulfilled with our career, happier with our marriage, or the parent of relatively self-controlled children. More than anything, we want to have less stress and more joy.

So why does it seem we can never quite get there? No matter how hard we try, it always seems to be just out of reach. We try all the latest and greatest diet tips, success strategies, marriage tips or parenting techniques, but things just don't seem to change. And all the trying is stressful and steals even more joy from us.

Why does it seem like we can never quite get to the life we've always wanted? It's probably that we set goals without having a specific plan of action for how to get there.

Goals are a good thing, but they aren't enough. Saying 'My goal is to have less stress and more joy' isn't going to work. It's too obscure. But it is attainable. In this combination journal/ planner which serves as a life change coach and accountability partner, Vicki will help you:

- Define what 'less stress' and 'more joy' means in your life

- Break your goals into manageable action steps

- Focus on progress rather than end goals

- Learn to continuously assess – Is what I'm doing right now getting me closer to where I want to be and to the person I want to become?

Join others on the Journey to Joy and let Vicki help you create the life you've always wanted.

9 780998 895413